Hiking In
Switzerland

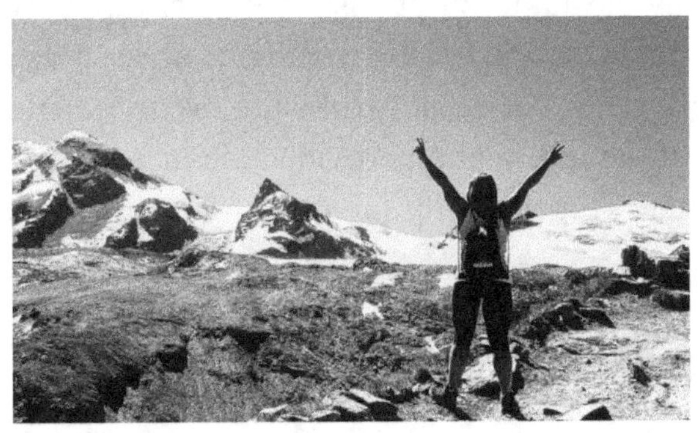

Detailed descriptions of trails, what to see, individual hike difficulties, route, distance, time and grade, where to sleep and eat, and more.

Kyle N. Wentz

Contents

Introduction

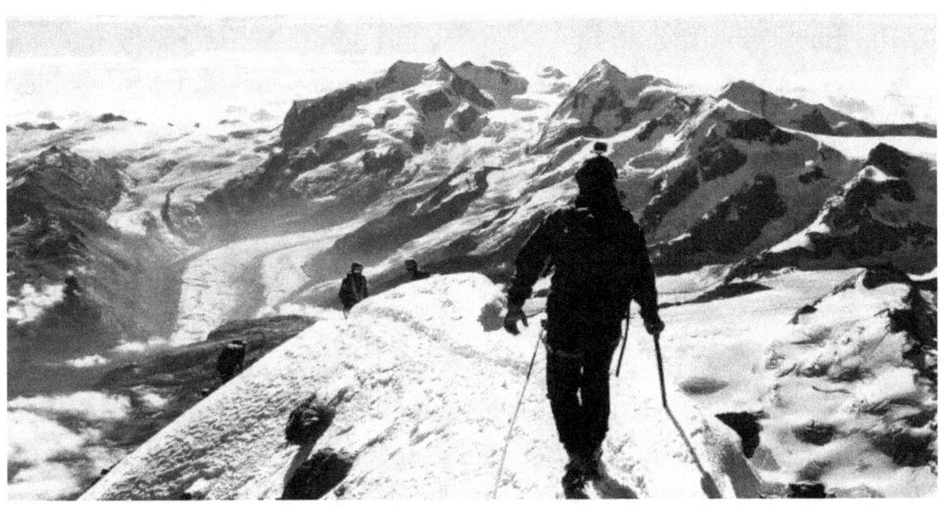

In the heart of Europe lies a hiker's haven, a place where the mountains rise with dignity and the valleys stretch with quiet grace. Switzerland, with its alpine splendor, offers a canvas of natural beauty that captivates the soul and ignites the wanderlust within.

As you set foot on Swiss soil, the grandeur of the Alps greets you, their peaks dusted with eternal snows that gleam like diamonds under the sun's gaze. The lakes, ever so clear, reflect the heavens above, creating a seamless blend of azure and emerald that soothes the eye and calms the mind.

The valleys, lush and fertile, are a testament to nature's nurturing hand, with wildflowers dotting the meadows in a riot of colors. The air, tinged with the scent of pine and the freshness of glacial streams, fills the lungs with purity, and each breath becomes a silent ode to the majesty of the mountains.

Switzerland's trails are not just routes through the wilderness; they are journeys through time and space. They whisper tales of ancient glaciers that sculpted the land, of forests that have stood sentinel for centuries, and of the delicate balance between man and nature that has been preserved with reverence.

The allure of these trails has been echoed by many famous hikers, their words a tribute to the transformative power of the Swiss landscape. "The mountains are not arenas where I satisfy my ambition to achieve," said the great climber Reinhold Messner, "they are the cathedrals where I practice my religion." And certainly, for those who walk these paths, the experience is nothing short of spiritual.

From the iconic Matterhorn, standing solitary and proud, to the serene shores of Lake Geneva, Switzerland's hiking trails invite you to explore, to discover, and to connect with the earth in a way that is both profound and personal.

As you ascend the rugged paths, the challenges of the climb are met with rewards beyond measure. The panoramic views that unfold from the mountain passes are scenes of such splendor that they seem painted by the hand of the divine. And in the quiet moments, when the wind carries the songs of the Alps and the distant call of an eagle, you find a peace that transcends the chaos of the world below.

The stories of those who have walked these trails before are etched into the very stones and streams. The laughter of children echoing in the valleys, the camaraderie of fellow hikers sharing a meal under the stars, and the silent communion with nature that speaks to the heart—these are the moments that define the Swiss hiking experience.

So let the call of the Swiss Alps beckon you to a world where beauty knows no bounds, where each step is a discovery, and where the journey itself becomes a cherished memory. For in Switzerland, every trail is an invitation to witness the harmony of nature, and every peak a testament to the enduring allure of the mountains.

And when the day's hike comes to an end, as you sit by the warmth of a fire, gazing at the stars that adorn the night sky, you realize that Switzerland has given you more than just a hike; it has given you a glimpse into the sublime, a touch of the infinite, and a sense of belonging to something greater than yourself.

This is the essence of Switzerland's hiking paradise—a place where the spirit soars, the heart finds joy, and the journey never truly ends

❖ Brief History

Switzerland has been a crossroads of cultures and a beacon of neutrality for centuries. Its history is as rich and varied as the landscapes that define it. From the early days when the Helvetii tribes roamed the valleys, to the Roman conquest that brought roads and cities, Switzerland has always been a place of movement and exchange.

The Middle Ages saw the rise of the Old Swiss Confederacy, a union of cantons that defied the might of empires and laid the groundwork for modern Switzerland. The spirit of independence and cooperation that characterized this period is still evident in the country's political structure today.

With the advent of the Reformation and the Enlightenment, Switzerland became a haven for thinkers and artists, its mountains and lakes providing inspiration and solace. It was during these times that the tradition of hiking began to take root in Swiss culture.

Hiking in Switzerland is not merely a pastime; it is a connection to the past. The trails that crisscross the nation are the same paths walked by pilgrims, traders, and soldiers throughout history. They are routes that have witnessed the passage of time and the footsteps of generations.

Among these historic trails is the Via Alpina, a path that traverses the entirety of the Swiss Alps, offering hikers a glimpse into the heart of this mountainous region. The Eiger Trail, with its proximity to the formidable north face of the Eiger mountain, provides a thrilling experience for those who walk its course.

The Gotthard Pass, once a vital trade route between northern and southern Europe, is now a popular hiking destination, its cobbled stones and ancient inns telling stories of the travelers who have passed this way.

The Aletsch Glacier trail allows hikers to witness the grandeur of the largest glacier in the Alps, a testament to the power of nature and the changing climate that shapes our world.

As you traverse these trails, you walk in the footsteps of history, each step a reminder of the enduring legacy of Switzerland. The act of hiking becomes an act of discovery, revealing not only the beauty of the landscape but also the layers of history that have shaped this nation.

In writing the history of Switzerland and its trails, one does not simply recount facts and dates; one weaves a narrative of resilience, community, and the timeless allure of the mountains. It is a story that continues to unfold with each hiker that sets out to explore the wonders of this remarkable country.

Changes over time

Hiking in Switzerland has undergone a remarkable transformation from its humble beginnings to the present day. Initially, the trails served practical purposes for locals, facilitating travel and commerce. As Switzerland's natural beauty gained international acclaim, these paths were enhanced to accommodate tourists seeking the Alpine allure.

The 1930s marked a pivotal era for Swiss hiking, with enthusiasts ensuring consistent signposting across the nation, simplifying navigation for hikers of varying expertise. Trails were categorized by difficulty, with yellow signs for easier routes and red-and-white for more challenging mountain trails. The rare blue-and-white signs point to alpine trails, often necessitating technical gear1.

Technological advancements have further refined the hiking experience. Today, hikers have access to detailed maps and online resources, providing current trail information.

Climate change has also left its mark on Swiss hiking. Melting glaciers have changed some trails, raising their difficulty and requiring greater environmental awareness from hikers1.

Now, Switzerland boasts over 65,000 km of marked trails, catering to a spectrum of preferences and abilities. From peaceful valley strolls to adventurous glacier treks, the growth of hiking in Switzerland ensures a rich and varied experience for every enthusiast

❖ Weather and Climate

Switzerland offers a climate as varied as its topography. The country's weather patterns are influenced by its geographical diversity, with the Alps playing a central role. To the north, the climate is more continental, with cold winters and warm summers, while the south enjoys a milder Mediterranean influence. This climatic dichotomy affects not only the daily life of its inhabitants but also the experiences of those who traverse its landscapes on foot.

The Alpine region, with its towering mountains, experiences a colder climate, where snow can persist even in the warmer months. Hikers venturing into these elevations must be prepared for sudden weather changes, as clear skies can swiftly give way to snowstorms. The pre-Alpine regions, however, offer a more temperate climate, ideal for those seeking a less arduous journey through nature's splendor.

As the seasons turn, so do the hiking conditions. The arrival of spring breathes life into the valleys, with snowmelt feeding the rivers and wildflowers beginning to dot the meadows. This period of renewal, however, can present challenges for hikers, as trails at higher altitudes may still be covered in snow or rendered impassable by the thaw.

Summer unveils the full glory of the Swiss landscape, with clear skies and stable weather providing optimal conditions for exploring the mountains. It is during these months that the high-altitude trails become accessible, revealing panoramic vistas and the vibrant hues of alpine flora.

Autumn casts a golden light on the hills, with cooler temperatures and fewer visitors making it a favored time for many to hit the trails. The lower elevations offer leisurely walks among the changing foliage, while the higher peaks may already see the first dustings of snow, signaling the approach of winter.

Winter transforms the Swiss Alps into a wonderland for snowshoeing and winter hiking, with well-groomed trails winding through the snow-covered landscape. It is a season of contrasts, where the stark beauty of the mountains is softened by the blanket of white.

For the hiking enthusiast, understanding these climate zones and their seasonal shifts is crucial. The best times for hiking are when nature is most stable—normally from late June to September, when the snow has exited to the highest peaks and the weather is most reliable. It is then that one can fully enjoy the harmony between climate and terrain, and the way they shape the Swiss hiking experience.

Flora and Fauna

There is an array of plants and animals that captivate the hearts of nature enthusiasts in Switzerland. The Swiss landscape, with its varying altitudes and climates, creates unique habitats for a diverse range of flora and fauna.

In the lower altitudes, the Swiss Plateau flourishes with deciduous forests where beech and oak trees dominate. As one ascends, coniferous trees such as spruce, fir, and larch become prevalent, painting the mountainside with hues of green. Among these wooded areas, one can find a variety of ferns, mosses, and wildflowers, including the rare and protected Lady's Slipper Orchid.

The alpine meadows burst into color during spring and summer, showcasing a spectacular display of wildflowers. The Edelweiss, Switzerland's national flower, is a symbol of the country's natural beauty and ruggedness. These meadows are also where one might spot the delicate Alpine Aster or the bold Alpine Rose.

Switzerland's wildlife is as varied as its plant life. The majestic ibex, with its impressive curved horns, roams the rocky crags of the Alps. The nimble chamois, a goat-antelope species, is equally at home in these high altitudes. Both species were once on the brink of extinction but have made remarkable comebacks thanks to conservation efforts.

Birdwatchers will delight in the variety of avian species that inhabit Switzerland. The Golden Eagle, with its awe-inspiring wingspan, soars above the mountain peaks, while the Nutcracker, a member of the crow family, is often heard before it's seen, thanks to its distinctive call. The Wallcreeper, with its crimson wings, clings to the vertical rock faces, and the Bearded Vulture, or Lammergeier, circles high in search of carrion.

Switzerland's commitment to conservation ensures that these natural wonders continue to thrive. The country's national parks and reserves protect the habitats of countless species, allowing visitors to experience the splendor of Swiss biodiversity. Whether one is traversing the Jura Mountains or exploring the valleys of the Alps, the encounter with Switzerland's flora and fauna is a profound reminder of the country's dedication to preserving its natural heritage.

As you hike the trails, keep your senses alert. The rustling leaves may reveal a Red Squirrel scurrying by, and the melodious song of the Alpine Chough may guide your path. Each step brings a discovery, a fresh wonder, and a deeper appreciation for the intricate tapestry of life that Switzerland so graciously hosts.

❖ Geography By Regions

Switzerland is divided into several distinct regions, each offering unique geographical features and hiking experiences.

Eastern Switzerland is characterized by its rolling hills and serene valleys. The region is home to the Appenzell Alps, where hikers can traverse through alpine meadows and past traditional Swiss chalets. The Säntis, the highest peak in the area, provides panoramic views that are simply awe-inspiring.

Zürich, the largest city in Switzerland, is surrounded by the lush Zürichsee and verdant hills. The Uetliberg mountain offers a quick escape from urban life, with trails leading to an overlook that presents the city and lake in all their glory.

Central Switzerland is the heart of the country, where legends and history intertwine. Lake Lucerne is flanked by mountains like Pilatus and Rigi, known as the "Queen of the Mountains," offering paths that wind through picturesque landscapes and reveal the history of the Swiss Confederation.

Northwestern Switzerland features the Jura Mountains, a range of limestone peaks stretching along the Swiss-French border. The Jura Crest Trail is a long-distance hike that rewards adventurers with views of the Rhine and the Black Forest.

Espace Mittelland is a region of contrast, with the Swiss Plateau's gentle topography giving way to the rugged Bernese Alps. The Emmental Valley, famous for its cheese, also boasts gentle hills ideal for leisurely hikes.

Ticino, the Italian-speaking region of Switzerland, is graced with a Mediterranean flair. The valleys of Verzasca, Maggia, and Ticino offer sunny skies and trails lined with palm trees, leading to clear, turquoise waters.

Région lémanique, bordering Lake Geneva, is a hiker's paradise with the terraced vineyards of Lavaux and the tranquil shores of the lake. The peaks of the Vaud Alps stand guard over the region, inviting hikers to explore their slopes.

The Swiss Alps, a majestic mountain range, are the backbone of Switzerland. Iconic peaks such as the Matterhorn and Eiger challenge experienced hikers, while the Aletsch Glacier, the largest in the Alps, is a testament to the awe-inspiring power of nature.

The Jura Mountains, with their densely forested landscapes, offer a stark contrast to the high Alps. The Doubs River carves through the region, creating opportunities for riverside hikes and exploration of the remote valleys.

The Swiss Plateau, stretching between the Jura and the Alps, is a patchwork of farmland, forests, and lakes. Trails here are perfect for those seeking a more relaxed hiking experience, with the chance to witness the daily life of Swiss villages.

Each region of Switzerland presents a unique chapter in the story of this country's geography, requesting hikers to discover its natural wonders and cultural richness. Whether scaling the heights of the Alps or wandering through the Jura's hidden valleys, Switzerland offers a world of adventure for every hiker.

Chapter 1

Know Before You Go

❖ When to Go

The question of when to visit this alpine wonderland for hiking is best answered by considering the interplay of weather patterns, visitor traffic, and the natural spectacle on display.

The Swiss hiking season unfurls its splendor starting in late spring, around May, when the lower valleys shed their winter chill, and the meadows begin to bloom with a riot of wildflowers. The air is crisp, the skies clear, and the trails less frequented, providing a serene setting for those seeking solitude alongside nature's awakening. Waterfalls, fed by melting snow, are at their most majestic, cascading with a roar that resonates through the valleys.

As June approaches, the higher altitudes start to become accessible. The lingering snowfields add a touch of drama to the rugged landscape, and the days grow longer, allowing more time to explore the extensive network of trails. This period is a delicate balance, with some higher routes still snowbound, while others beckon with clear paths and panoramic views.

The peak of summer, from July to September, is the golden window for hikers in Switzerland. The high alpine routes are clear of snow, revealing paths that weave through verdant pastures, skirt crystal-clear lakes, and traverse beneath towering peaks. The weather is warm, yet the altitude offers a reprieve from the heat, with the occasional afternoon thunderstorm to cool the air and amplify the alpine glow of sunsets.

This season also coincides with the busiest time for tourism. Trails around famous landmarks can be bustling, but with the vastness of the Swiss Alps, one can always find a quieter corner to enjoy. It's a time of vibrant alpine culture, with local festivities and the sound of cowbells echoing across the hills, adding a rhythmic backdrop to the hiker's journey.

Autumn casts a different spell on the Swiss landscape. From October, the crowds dissipate, and the forests don a fiery mantle of reds, oranges, and golds. The air turns sharp, signaling the approach of winter, but for those who venture out, the crisp atmosphere offers unparalleled clarity for viewing the distant peaks. It's a reflective time, perfect for those who appreciate the melancholic beauty of nature's preparations for the snowy blanket to come.

Winter hiking in Switzerland has its charm, with a selection of trails specially groomed for the season. January and February are ideal for those who enjoy the crunch of snow underfoot and the silence of a winter wonderland. The landscape transforms into a realm of purity, where the starkness of snow-covered peaks contrasts with the deep blues of the sky.

Ultimately, the best time to hike in Switzerland truly depends on what one seeks from the experience. Whether it's the fresh vitality of spring, the exuberance of summer, the contemplative calm of autumn, or the serene stillness of winter, Switzerland's trails offer year-round allure. Each season paints the mountains with a different brush, inviting hikers to step into a living canvas that evolves with time. The key is to choose the season that resonates with your spirit and step onto the trails with an open heart, ready to embrace the adventure that awaits.

❖ What to Bring

In preparation for these diverse seasonal offerings, hikers must equip themselves appropriately. The right gear can make the difference between a trek that's merely memorable and one that's truly transformative. Here's a comprehensive checklist to ensure you're well-equipped for y**our Swiss adventure.**

Clothing Layers: The Swiss climate can be as varied as its topography, so layering is key. Begin with a moisture-wicking base coating that keeps you dry. Add a mid-layer, such as a fleece or down jacket, that insulates and retains body heat. Top it off with a waterproof and windproof shell layer to protect against the elements. Don't forget thermal leggings for those cooler altitudes.

Footwear: Your feet are your most valuable asset on the trail. Choose waterproof, breathable hiking boots with good ankle support and grip. Break them in well before your journey to avoid blisters. Pack several pairs of wool or synthetic socks to keep your feet dry and cushioned.

Navigation Tools: A reliable map and compass are indispensable for navigating the Swiss trails. Consider a GPS device or a smartphone with a GPS app, but remember that technology can fail, so get a physical map as a backup.

Safety Items: Safety should never be an afterthought. Include a first-aid kit tailored to your group's needs, a multi-tool with a knife, and a whistle for emergencies. A headlamp or flashlight with extra batteries is essential, as daylight can be unpredictable. Sun protection, including sunscreen, sunglasses, and a hat, will shield you from UV rays at higher elevations.

Supplies: Hydration is crucial. Carry a water bottle or hydration system, and know the locations of water sources along your route. Pack high-energy snacks like parched fruit, nuts, and energy bars. For longer treks, add dehydrated meals that only require hot water.

Additional Gear: Trekking poles can reduce the impact on your knees and improve balance. A lightweight, durable backpack with a rain cover will protect your gear. Don't forget a camera to capture the breathtaking vistas, and consider binoculars for wildlife spotting.

Remember, the key to a successful hike is not just what you bring, but also what you leave behind. Pack light, choose multipurpose items, and prepare for the unexpected. With this checklist, you'll be ready to embrace the Swiss mountains with confidence and comfort.

Preparing for a Hike and Emergency Procedures

Hiking in Switzerland is an experience that captures the heart and soul of every adventurer. The majestic mountains, serene lakes, and charming villages make it a paradise for hikers. But, as with any tale, preparation is key.

Physical fitness is the cornerstone of a successful hike. Regular cardiovascular exercises such as running, cycling, or swimming can help build stamina. Strength training, particularly for the legs and core, is also essential. Remember, the Swiss Alps are not just beautiful; they are also challenging.

Mental preparation is equally important. Enlighten yourself with the trail map and weather situations. Learn about the flora and fauna. Understand the culture and customs of the local communities. This knowledge will not only enrich your hiking experience but also help you respect the environment and local traditions.

Setting realistic expectations is crucial. Not every day will be sunny, and not every trail will be easy. There may be times when you'll have to turn back or change your plans. That's okay. The mountains aren't going anywhere. It's better to be safe and enjoy the journey than to push yourself too hard and risk injury.

Now, let's talk about emergency procedures. Accidents can occur, even to the most professional hikers. That's why knowing basic first aid is a must.

Cardiopulmonary resuscitation, or CPR, can be a lifesaver. If a person is unconscious and not breathing, start chest compressions immediately. Push hard and quickly in the middle of the chest, at a speed of 100 to 120 compressions per minute. If you're trained, give rescue breaths after every 30 compressions.

Bleeding is another common hiking injury. If someone is bleeding, apply pressure to the wound with a clean bandage or cloth. If possible, elevate the wound. If the bleeding doesn't cease, seek medical help instantly.

Recognizing signs of distress is also important. Symptoms like dizziness, confusion, rapid heartbeat, and shortness of breath could indicate a serious condition like heat stroke or hypothermia. If you notice these signs, stop, rest, hydrate, and seek help if necessary.

Remember, safety should always be your top priority. Equip yourself with the right knowledge and skills, respect the mountains, and they will reward you with an unforgettable experience.

❖ Permits, Regulations and Trail Etiquette

From the serene valleys to the challenging Alpine ascents, each hiking path in Switzerland presents a unique encounter with nature. However, to ensure the preservation of this natural splendor and the safety of all adventurers, it is crucial to adhere to the country's hiking regulations and obtain the necessary permits.

The Swiss take great pride in their hiking infrastructure, meticulously maintained by the Swiss Hiking Trail Federation. The trails are marked with precision, indicating the difficulty level and estimated time to reach various points of interest. For the casual wanderer, trails marked with yellow signs promise a leisurely experience, while the more daring can follow the red-and-white or blue-and-white signs for a taste of the Alpine challenge.

When planning an excursion into the Swiss wilderness, one must be aware of the specific permits required for certain regions. For instance, hiking in national parks or nature reserves often necessitates a permit, which serves as a commitment to respect the environment and its inhabitants. These permits are not mere formalities; they are a pledge to uphold the sanctity of these protected areas.

In Switzerland, the harmony between humans and wildlife is of utmost importance. Regulations are in place to protect the diverse species that call the mountains home. Hikers are expected to maintain a respectful distance from animals, refrain from feeding them, and adhere to designated paths to minimize disturbance.

Camping in Switzerland is a magical experience, yet it comes with its own set of rules. Wild camping is generally prohibited, especially in protected areas. Designated camping sites are available, providing the necessary amenities while ensuring minimal impact on the environment.

The Swiss trails are a marvel of meticulous maintenance, with 65,000 km of marked paths that promise safe and enjoyable adventures. The

Swiss Hiking Trail Federation, along with local communities, has established a set of unwritten rules that foster mutual respect and minimize the impact on the environment.

Greeting fellow hikers with a simple "Grüezi" or a nod is a customary practice that adds a touch of warmth to the journey. It's a small gesture that acknowledges the shared passion for the great outdoors and creates a sense of camaraderie among hikers.

Yielding the trail is a practical aspect of trail etiquette. When encountering others, the general rule is that those ascending have the right of way. This courtesy allows for a smoother flow of traffic and prevents bottlenecks on narrow paths.

Minimizing one's impact on the environment is paramount. Staying on marked trails protects the surrounding flora and prevents soil erosion. Hikers are encouraged to carry out what they carry in, leaving no trace of their presence. This practice ensures that the natural beauty of the Swiss landscape remains unspoiled for future visitors.

Responsible behavior extends to interactions with wildlife. Observing animals from a distance without disturbing their natural habitat is essential. Feeding wildlife is discouraged as it can alter their behavior and diet.

The Swiss ethos of respect for nature is embodied in every regulation. By adhering to these regulations, hikers play a vital role in the conservation efforts that safeguard Switzerland's natural heritage. The permits and guidelines are not merely bureaucratic hurdles but are integral to maintaining the integrity of the country's hiking culture. They reflect a collective commitment to environmental stewardship and responsible tourism.

❖ Essential Tips for Hiking in Switzerland

To ensure a memorable and safe hiking adventure, here are some essential tips, along with insights into the cultural nuances and local customs that will enrich your journey.

Preparation is Key Before setting out, it's crucial to plan your route carefully. Switzerland boasts a well-maintained network of trails, with clear signage and difficulty ratings. Select a trail that fits your fitness level and experience. Check the weather forecast, as mountain conditions can change rapidly, and always inform someone about your itinerary.

Gear Up Appropriately Invest in quality hiking boots that provide good ankle support and grip. Dress in layers to adapt to changing temperatures, and don't forget a waterproof jacket. A backpack with essentials such as water, snacks, a map, a compass, and a first-aid kit is a must. Consider a hiking pole for additional stability.

Respect the Environment Switzerland is known for its pristine natural landscapes. Stick to marked trails to avoid damaging the flora and fauna. Carry out all your trash, and be mindful of noise levels, as the tranquility of the mountains is cherished by both locals and wildlife.

Understand the Grading System Swiss trails are graded according to difficulty: yellow for easy, red and white for medium, and blue for challenging. Respect these gradings, as they are there for your safety.

Timing Your Hike Start early to make the most of daylight hours and avoid afternoon thunderstorms, which are common in the Alps. Allow ample time to complete your hike without rushing, as this increases the risk of accidents.

Safety First Always check the condition of the trails with local tourist offices or mountain guides. Avalanches and rockfalls are real dangers, so heed any warnings and restrictions. Consider hiring a local guide if you're venturing into more challenging terrain.

Cultural Insights Switzerland has four official languages: German, French, Italian, and Romansh. Greeting fellow hikers with a simple "Grüezi," "Bonjour," or "Buongiorno" can go a long way in showing respect. Swiss people value punctuality, so if you've arranged a guided hike or a group meet-up, be on time.

Local Customs Mountain huts and alpine restaurants are great places to rest and refuel. It's customary to share tables with strangers due to limited space. When doing so, a polite greeting is appreciated. Tipping is not mandatory, but rounding up the bill is a common practice.

Celebrate the Alpine Culture Participate in local festivals and events if your visit coincides with them. These celebrations are a fantastic way to experience Swiss traditions, music, and cuisine.

Insurance and Rescue Services Ensure you have appropriate insurance that covers mountain rescue services. In case of an emergency, the universal European emergency number is 112.

❖ Choosing the Right Trail

Choosing the right trail in Switzerland can be a delightful experience, filled with stunning vistas, diverse terrain, and the opportunity to connect deeply with nature. The process of selecting the perfect trail involves thoughtful consideration of your personal preferences, fitness level, hiking experience, trail lengths, and seasonal factors. Let's dive into these aspects to ensure your hiking adventure in Switzerland is both enjoyable and memorable.

First and foremost, personal preferences play a significant role in determining which trail to choose. Switzerland offers a vast array of hiking options, from gentle walks through pastoral valleys to challenging ascents up rugged mountain paths. Think about what kind of scenery you most enjoy. Do you prefer tranquil lakes and verdant forests, or are you more drawn to the dramatic peaks and high-altitude panoramas? Perhaps you enjoy exploring cultural landmarks and quaint villages along the way, or maybe the allure of remote wilderness appeals to your sense of adventure. Understanding your preferences helps narrow down the plethora of options to those that will most satisfy your interests and provide the kind of experience you are seeking.

Your fitness level is another crucial factor to consider. Hiking can be a strenuous activity, and the diverse topography of Switzerland means that trails can vary widely in terms of difficulty. Beginners and those looking for a more leisurely experience might opt for trails with minimal elevation gain and shorter distances. These might include routes like the walk around Lake Lucerne or the easy path from Zermatt to Zmutt, which offer beautiful views without demanding too much physically. For the more physically fit and experienced hikers, challenging trails such as the Eiger Trail, which requires a good level of endurance and involves significant elevation changes, might be more appropriate. It's important to be honest with yourself about your fitness level to ensure that your hike is safe and enjoyable.

Experience in hiking is another important consideration. If you are new to hiking, starting with well-marked and popular trails can provide a sense of security and ease. These trails often have amenities such as rest stops, clear signage, and sometimes even guided options. The Five Lakes Walk near Zermatt is an excellent choice for novices, offering clear paths and spectacular views of the Matterhorn reflected in the lakes. Experienced hikers, on the other hand, might seek out more remote and challenging trails, such as the Via Alpina, which traverses the entire country from east to west, offering a more rugged and solitary experience.

Trail length is another key element in choosing the right hike. Day hikes are perfect for those who want to enjoy the beauty of Switzerland without committing to an overnight stay. Trails such as the Lauterbrunnen Valley walk, which can be completed in a few hours, offer stunning scenery and can be easily fitted into a day's itinerary. For those looking for a more immersive experience, multi-day hikes like the Haute Route from Chamonix to Zermatt provide a more extensive adventure, requiring careful planning and perhaps staying in mountain huts or local inns along the way. Consider how much time you have and how long you are comfortable hiking each day when selecting your trail.

Seasonal considerations are also paramount when planning your hike in Switzerland. The hiking season typically runs from late spring to early autumn, with the best conditions usually found between June and September. During these months, trails are generally clear of snow, weather conditions are more stable, and mountain huts and other amenities are open. Spring hikes can offer the beauty of blooming wildflowers and fewer crowds, but some higher-altitude trails may still be snow-covered and challenging to navigate. Autumn hikes provide a spectacular display of changing foliage, with cooler temperatures making for comfortable hiking conditions. However, it's important to note that weather in the mountains can change rapidly, and trails may become slippery with early snowfall. Winter hiking is a different experience altogether, often requiring special equipment such as snowshoes and a good knowledge of avalanche risks.

To summarize, choosing the right trail in Switzerland involves a balance of several factors. Start with your personal preferences, considering what kind of scenery and experiences most appeal to you. Evaluate your fitness level honestly, ensuring you choose a trail that matches your physical capabilities. Consider your hiking experience, opting for well-marked and popular trails if you are a beginner, or seeking out more remote and challenging paths if you are experienced. Think about how much time you have and how long you want to hike, selecting a trail length that fits your schedule and stamina. Finally, take into account the season, aiming to hike during the optimal months of late spring to early autumn, and always being prepared for changing weather conditions.

❖ Getting to Switzerland

Getting to this picturesque country is straightforward, thanks to its well-connected airports and efficient transportation network. Here's everything you need to know about traveling to Switzerland, including airports, direct flights, travel times, visas, immigration, luggage claims, flight comparison websites, flight prices, car hire, connecting flights, airport facilities, currency exchange, and transportation from the airport to the city center.

Switzerland is served by several major international airports. Zurich Airport, the largest and busiest, is situated in the northern part of the country and offers numerous direct flights from major cities worldwide. Geneva Airport, located near the French border, is another major hub with extensive international connections. Basel-Mulhouse-Freiburg Airport, uniquely positioned near the tripoint of Switzerland, France, and Germany, also provides a variety of direct flights. For those flying into the capital, Bern Airport offers limited but efficient connections, mainly serving European destinations.

Direct flights to Switzerland are plentiful, making it accessible from numerous global locations. For example, a flight from New York to Zurich takes approximately eight hours, while London to Geneva is a quick one-and-a-half-hour journey. From Dubai to Zurich, expect a travel time of around seven hours, and for those coming from Sydney, the journey to Zurich typically takes about 24 hours with one stop. Major airlines such as Swiss International Air Lines, British Airways, Lufthansa, Emirates, and United Airlines frequently operate direct flights to Switzerland, ensuring a variety of options for travelers.

Upon arrival, passengers will go through immigration control. Having your passport and, if necessary, a visa ready for inspection will expedite the process. Swiss airports are known for their efficiency, so the immigration process is usually swift. After clearing immigration, proceed to the luggage claim area, which is well-signposted and equipped with free luggage carts. Should you encounter any issues with your luggage, the lost and found counters staffed by airport personnel are there to assist.

Planning your trip can be more budget-friendly by comparing flight prices across various platforms. Websites such as Skyscanner, Kayak, Momondo, and Google Flights are excellent resources for finding the best deals. The cost of flights to Switzerland varies depending on the season, airline, and how far in advance you book. Typically, round-trip fares from the United States range from $500 to $1,500. Within Europe, round-trip tickets can be as low as $100, particularly with budget airlines.

For those who prefer the freedom of exploring by car, renting a vehicle at the airport is a convenient option. Zurich, Geneva, Basel, and Bern airports all feature a range of car rental agencies, including Hertz, Avis, Europcar, Sixt, and Enterprise. Car rental desks are usually located in the arrivals hall or a designated car rental center, making it easy to pick up your vehicle shortly after landing. It's advisable to book your car in advance to secure the best rates and ensure availability. When renting a car, you will need to present your driver's license, passport, and credit card. For those planning to drive extensively, renting a GPS can be incredibly helpful for navigation.

If direct flights aren't available from your departure city, connecting flights through major European hubs like Frankfurt, Paris Charles de Gaulle, Amsterdam Schiphol, and London Heathrow are excellent alternatives. These airports offer frequent flights to Switzerland, ensuring a smooth and convenient travel experience.

To find the best flights, booking early is essential, as flight prices tend to rise closer to the departure date. Flexibility with travel dates can also help you find lower fares. Using price alert features on comparison websites to monitor fare changes and considering flights into nearby airports with onward travel by train or bus can sometimes result in significant savings.

Swiss airports are equipped with top-notch facilities to ensure a comfortable travel experience. Free Wi-Fi is available throughout the airports, letting you stay connected. Various lounges offer a relaxing environment, some with shower facilities to refresh after a long flight. Dining options are plentiful, ranging from quick snacks to full meals, and duty-free shops offer a variety of products at tax-free prices. Medical assistance is also available in case of crises.

Currency exchange services are readily available at Swiss airports, with multiple counters and ATMs where you can withdraw Swiss Francs (CHF). While exchanging currency at the airport is convenient, it's worth noting that the exchange rates may not be as favorable as those at banks or local exchange offices in the city.

Transportation from Swiss airports to city centers is seamless, thanks to the country's highly efficient public transportation system. From Zurich Airport, the quickest and most convenient option to reach Zurich city center is by train. Trains run frequently and take about 10-15 minutes to reach Zurich Hauptbahnhof, the main train station. The airport also connects to the city via tram line 10, which takes around 35 minutes. Taxis are available outside the arrivals hall and take approximately 20 minutes to the city center, though they are more expensive than public transport.

Geneva Airport also offers excellent connectivity to the city center. Trains to Geneva's main station run every 10-15 minutes, with a travel time of about seven minutes. Several bus lines connect the airport to various parts of the city, taking around 20 minutes. Taxis are available and take about 15 minutes to the city center.

Basel-Mulhouse-Freiburg Airport connects to Basel city center via the Airport Bus Line 50, which runs frequently to Basel's main train station, with a journey time of about 20 minutes. Taxis are also available and take approximately 15 minutes to reach the city center.

For those arriving at Bern Airport, the easiest way to reach Bern city center is by bus line 334, which connects the airport to Belp, where you can transfer to a train to Bern. The total journey takes around 30 minutes. Taxis are available and take about 20 minutes to the city center.

❖ Local Transport

Traveling through Switzerland is a pleasure thanks to its extensive and highly efficient public transportation network. From sleek trains to scenic ferries, Switzerland offers various options to get you from point A to point B with ease. Let's take a detailed look at the different modes of transportation available, including the companies that operate them, ticket prices, passes, routes, stations, operation hours, and tips for using taxis.

Swiss Federal Railways (SBB)

The backbone of Switzerland's public transport is the Swiss Federal Railways (SBB), which operates an extensive network of trains connecting cities, towns, and even remote areas. The trains are known for their punctuality, cleanliness, and comfort. Major routes include Zurich to Geneva, Bern to Interlaken, and Zurich to Lucerne. High-speed trains like the InterCity (IC) and EuroCity (EC) make long-distance travel quick and convenient.

Regional Trains

Regional trains, operated by various regional rail companies, serve smaller towns and rural areas. These trains connect seamlessly with the SBB network, making it easy to reach virtually any destination in Switzerland. They are especially useful for accessing hiking trails, ski resorts, and other outdoor activities. The SBB operates an extensive network that covers the entire country, connecting major cities, towns, and remote villages.

For example, a journey from Zurich to Geneva takes about three hours and costs approximately 75 CHF for a second-class ticket and 125 CHF for a first-class ticket. Tickets can be purchased at train stations, online via the SBB website, or through the SBB mobile app. The SBB app is particularly useful for checking timetables, purchasing tickets, and receiving real-time travel updates.

In addition to regular trains, Switzerland offers scenic routes such as the Glacier Express, which travels between Zermatt and St. Moritz, offering spectacular views of the Swiss Alps. Another popular route is the Bernina Express, which runs from Chur to Tirano, crossing the picturesque Alps and showcasing stunning landscapes.

Buses

Swiss cities and towns are well-served by buses, providing reliable connections to areas not accessible by train. PostBus Switzerland is the largest bus company, known for its distinctive yellow coaches.

PostBuses connect rural regions and alpine areas, often traveling through some of the most scenic parts of the country.

A typical bus fare for a short journey within a city costs around 2.50 to 4.00 CHF, depending on the distance. Tickets can be bought from ticket machines at bus stops, online, or via mobile apps. Multi-ride tickets and day passes are also available, offering convenience and savings for frequent travelers.

Trams

Trams are a vital part of public transportation in Swiss cities such as Zurich, Basel, Geneva, and Bern. Zurich's tram network is one of the most extensive, providing frequent service throughout the city and its suburbs. A single ticket for a short journey within Zurich costs 4.40 CHF, and it's valid for 60 minutes, allowing unlimited transfers within the city zones. Tickets can be purchased at tram stops, online, or via the ZVV app.

Tram operation hours typically start around 5 AM and run until midnight, with night services available on weekends. The Zurich Card, available for 24 or 72 hours, offers unlimited travel on Zurich's public transport, as well as discounts on city attractions.

Ferries

Switzerland's many lakes provide the perfect setting for ferry travel. Companies like the Lake Geneva General Navigation Company (CGN) operate ferries on major lakes such as Lake Geneva, Lake Zurich, and

Lake Lucerne. These ferries are not just a mode of transport but also offer a scenic way to explore the country.

A typical ferry ride on Lake Geneva, such as the route between Geneva and Montreux, costs around 25 CHF for a one-way trip. Tickets can be purchased at ferry terminals or online. The Swiss Travel Pass covers ferry rides, making it an excellent option for tourists.

Taxis

Taxis are readily available in Swiss cities and towns, though they can be expensive. Licensed taxis have a taxi sign on the roof and a meter inside the vehicle. To ensure you're getting a licensed taxi, look for the driver's ID and the meter. Taxis can be hailed on the street, booked via phone, or through mobile apps like Uber, which operates in some Swiss cities.

Taxi fares in Switzerland start at about 6 CHF, with an additional 3.50 CHF per kilometer. Tipping is not mandatory, but it's customary to round up the fare or add a small amount for good service. Bargaining is not a common practice in Switzerland.

Cable Cars and Funiculars

To access the high alpine regions, Switzerland has an extensive network of cable cars, funiculars, and cogwheel trains. These modes of transport are essential for reaching ski resorts, hiking trails, and mountain peaks. Notable examples include the Gornergrat Railway in Zermatt, which offers spectacular views of the Matterhorn, and the Jungfrau Railway, which takes you to the Jungfraujoch, known as the "Top of Europe."

Passes and Tickets

For tourists, the Swiss Travel Pass offers unlimited travel on the SBB network, most trams, buses, boats, and some mountain railways and cable cars. The pass is available for durations of 3, 4, 8, or 15 consecutive days and includes free entry to many museums and attractions. Prices for the Swiss Travel Pass start at 232 CHF for three days in second class.

Another option is the Swiss Half Fare Card, which allows travelers to purchase tickets for trains, buses, trams, and boats at half price. The card costs 120 CHF and is valid for one month.

Stations and Operation Hours

Swiss train stations are well-equipped with amenities such as ticket counters, self-service machines, shops, restaurants, and restrooms. Major stations like Zurich Hauptbahnhof, Geneva Cornavin, and Bern offer extensive facilities, including luggage storage, currency exchange, and tourist information centers.

Train and bus services typically start around 5 AM and run until midnight, with night services available on weekends in major cities. Always check the timetable for the specific route you plan to take, as operation hours may vary.

Overall Transportation Experience

Traveling by public transport in Switzerland is a seamless experience, known for its reliability and efficiency. The integration of trains, buses, trams, and ferries ensures that you can reach even the most remote corners of the country with ease. Whether you're traveling through the bustling cities, picturesque villages, or the majestic Alps, Swiss public transport offers a comfortable and scenic way to explore the country.

Car Rentals

To fully experience the beauty and reach the most secluded trails, renting a car is an excellent option. This guide provides all the information you need to navigate car rentals in Switzerland, from choosing the right rental company to understanding costs, requirements, and insurance options.

Choosing the Right Rental Company

Switzerland boasts several reputable car rental companies, each offering a range of vehicles to suit your needs. Major international firms like Hertz, Europcar, and Avis have a strong presence, providing reliable service and extensive networks. Hertz offers competitive pricing and a broad selection of vehicles, from compact cars perfect for city driving to larger SUVs suitable for mountain terrain. Their offices can be found in major cities such as Zurich, Geneva, and Basel, making it convenient to pick up and drop off your rental.

Europcar is another popular choice, known for its excellent customer service and diverse fleet. Their luxury car options are ideal for those seeking a more comfortable and stylish ride through the Swiss countryside. Avis also offers a similar range of vehicles, with a strong focus on customer satisfaction and flexible rental terms.

For more localized services, Swiss companies like Sixt and Mobility. Sixt, known for its affordable rates and wide selection of vehicles, is ideal for budget-conscious travelers. Mobility offers a unique car-sharing service, allowing you to rent cars by the hour or day, providing great flexibility for short trips or spontaneous hikes.

Types of Cars Available

When choosing a car, consider the type of terrain and weather conditions you'll encounter. Compact cars are perfect for city driving and shorter trips. They are easy to park and fuel-efficient, making them a cost-effective choice. For those planning to venture into the mountains or explore remote hiking trails, an SUV or a four-wheel-drive vehicle is recommended. These cars offer better stability and handling on uneven roads and in adverse weather conditions.

Luxury cars are available for those who prefer a more comfortable and stylish journey. These vehicles often come equipped with advanced features such as GPS navigation, which can be particularly useful when exploring unfamiliar areas.

Understanding Costs

The cost of renting a car in Switzerland can vary significantly depending on the type of vehicle, rental duration, and the rental company. On average, expect to pay between CHF 60 to CHF 150 per day for a standard car. Luxury vehicles and SUVs typically cost more, ranging from CHF 150 to CHF 400 per day.

Additional costs to consider include fuel, which is relatively expensive in Switzerland, and tolls for using certain highways. Some rental companies offer unlimited mileage, while others may charge extra if you exceed a certain distance. Be sure to clarify these details when booking your car.

Rental Requirements

To rent a car in Switzerland, you must be at least 20 years old, although some companies may require drivers to be 25 or older. A valid driver's license from your home country is generally sufficient, but it's advisable to carry an International Driving Permit (IDP) as well. Most rental companies require a credit card for the security deposit and payment.

When collecting your rental car, you will need to present your driver's license, passport, and the credit card used for the booking. It's important to inspect the car thoroughly before driving away, noting any existing damage to avoid disputes later.

Insurance Options

Car rental companies in Switzerland offer various insurance options to protect you in case of accidents or damage. Basic insurance, which includes Collision Damage Waiver (CDW) and Theft Protection, is usually included in the rental price. CDW reduces your financial liability in case of an accident, while Theft Protection covers the cost if the car is stolen.

Additional coverage, such as Super Collision Damage Waiver (SCDW) and Personal Accident Insurance (PAI), is available at an extra cost. SCDW further reduces your liability in case of an accident, and PAI provides medical coverage for injuries sustained in an accident. It's advisable to carefully review the terms and conditions of the insurance policies to ensure you have adequate coverage.

Rental Locations and Contact Information

Major Swiss cities and airports have numerous car rental offices, making it convenient to pick up and drop off your rental car. In Zurich, you can find rental offices at the airport (Flughafen Zürich, 8058 Zürich-Flughafen, +41 43 816 32 00 for Hertz) and the main train station (Bahnhofplatz 15, 8001 Zürich, +41 44 215 44 66 for Europcar). Geneva offers similar options, with rental offices at the airport (Route de l'Aéroport 21, 1215 Genève, +41 22 717 86 20 for Avis) and the train station (Rue de Lausanne 37, 1201 Genève, +41 22 901 12 40 for Sixt).

In Basel, car rentals are available at the EuroAirport (Aéroport de Bâle-Mulhouse, 68304 Saint-Louis, +33 3 89 90 22 20 for Europcar) and the central train station (Centralbahnstrasse 10, 4051 Basel, +41 61 365 90 00 for Hertz). Lucerne and Interlaken, popular starting points for hiking adventures, also have rental offices in their city centers.

Renting a car in Switzerland offers the freedom and flexibility to explore the country's breathtaking landscapes at your own pace. Whether you're planning a leisurely drive through picturesque villages or an adventurous trek in the Alps, the right rental car will enhance your Swiss hiking experience.

❖ Accommodation Options

When it comes to accommodation in Switzerland, hikers are spoilt for choice with a range of options to suit every preference and budget. Whether you prefer the comfort of a hotel, the charm of a guesthouse, or the camaraderie of a mountain hut, Switzerland offers something for everyone.

Hotels are a popular choice for many travelers, offering a range of amenities to ensure a comfortable stay. From cozy family-run establishments to luxurious five-star resorts, hotels in Switzerland come in all shapes and sizes. Most offer private rooms with ensuite bathrooms, as well as additional amenities such as restaurants, spas, and fitness facilities. Prices vary depending on the location and level of luxury, with options to suit every budget. Many hotels are conveniently located near popular hiking trails, providing easy access to the great outdoors. To reach them, travelers can often rely on public transportation, with many hotels offering shuttle services from nearby train stations or airports. Booking a hotel room in Switzerland is typically straightforward, with online booking platforms offering a convenient way to secure your accommodation in advance.

For those seeking a more intimate and authentic experience, guesthouses and bed and breakfasts are an excellent option. These charming establishments are often family-owned and operated, providing personalized service and a warm welcome to guests. Accommodation ranges from simple rooms with shared facilities to more spacious suites with private bathrooms. Prices are generally more affordable than hotels, making guesthouses a popular choice for budget-conscious travelers. Many guesthouses are located in picturesque villages and towns, with easy access to nearby hiking trails. Travelers can reach them by train, bus, or car, with parking available at most establishments. Booking a room in a guesthouse is often done directly with the property owners, either by phone or email.

For those looking to immerse themselves in nature, mountain huts offer a unique accommodation experience in Switzerland. These rustic lodgings are situated in remote locations high in the mountains, providing shelter and basic amenities to hikers and climbers. Accommodation is typically in dormitory-style rooms with shared facilities, and meals are often included in the price of the stay. Prices vary depending on the location and facilities available, with some mountain huts offering more comfort than others. Many huts are located along popular hiking routes, providing a convenient place to rest and refuel after a day on the trails. Access to mountain huts is usually on foot, with hiking being the only way to reach them. Booking a stay in a mountain hut is essential, especially during the busy summer months, and reservations can often be made online or by phone.

No matter what type of accommodation you choose, rest assured that Switzerland offers a range of options to suit every taste and budget. From luxurious hotels to charming guest houses to rustic mountain huts, there's something for everyone to enjoy. With convenient access to hiking trails, stunning natural scenery, and warm Swiss hospitality, your accommodation in Switzerland is sure to enhance your hiking experience.

Price Range

Prices can vary widely depending on factors such as location, amenities, and seasonality.

For hotels, prices typically range from around $100 to $500 per night for standard rooms, with luxury properties charging upwards of $500 or more. Budget options such as hostels or simpler hotels can sometimes be found for less than $100 per night.

Guesthouses and bed and breakfasts tend to offer more affordable rates, with prices ranging from $50 to $200 per night depending on the level of comfort and amenities provided.

Mountain huts, being more basic, generally offer the most economical accommodation options. Prices for a night's stay in a dormitory-style room with shared facilities can range from $20 to $100 per person, with meals sometimes included in the price.

It's important to keep in mind that these are estimated prices and actual rates may vary depending on factors such as location, time of booking, and special promotions. Additionally, prices in popular tourist destinations or during peak season may be higher.

Easy Trails (Perfect for Families and Beginners)

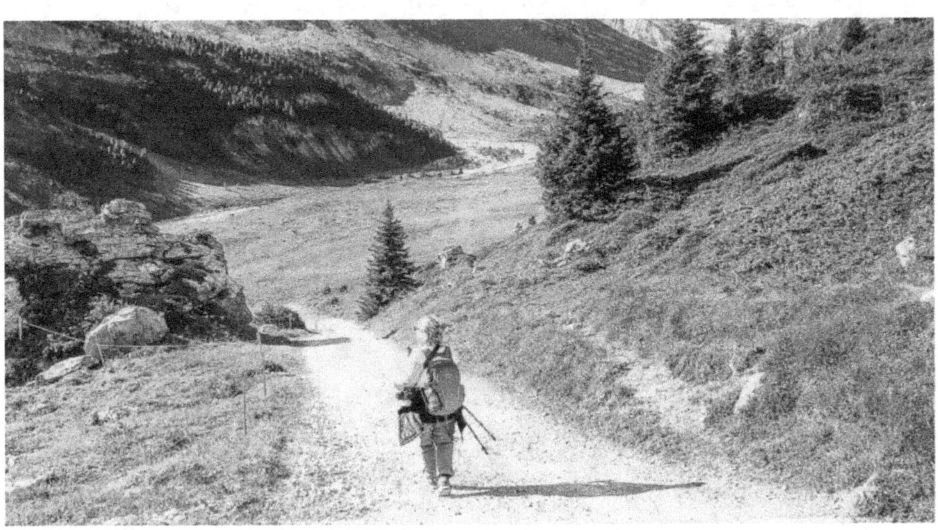

Lake Geneva Trail

The Lake Geneva Trail, also known as the Sentier du Lac Léman, is a captivating hike that offers a delightful mix of natural beauty, diverse wildlife, and rich historical features. Stretching along the northern shore of Lake Geneva, this trail provides an accessible and enjoyable adventure for hikers of all levels. Let's dive into the details that make this trail a must-experience for outdoor enthusiasts.

Starting from the city of Geneva and winding its way through picturesque towns like Nyon, Lausanne, and Montreux, the Lake Geneva Trail offers an unparalleled lakeside experience. The trail covers a total distance of approximately 200 kilometers (about 124 miles). Given the length, hikers often tackle the trail in segments, making it suitable for day hikes or extended trips.

The terrain of the Lake Geneva Trail is mostly flat to gently rolling, making it an accessible hike for most fitness levels. The altitude ranges from about 372 meters (1,220 feet) at the lakeside to a few hundred meters higher in some areas, providing a comfortable gradient for walking without any strenuous climbs. The trail is well-marked, with clear signage throughout, ensuring that hikers can easily follow the route without difficulty.

One of the highlights of the Lake Geneva Trail is the stunning variety of flora and fauna you'll encounter along the way. The lakeside environment supports a rich array of plant life, from lush vineyards that produce the region's famous wines to vibrant wildflowers that dot the path in spring and summer. Trees such as chestnut, oak, and maple provide shade and a sense of serenity as you walk. Wildlife enthusiasts will enjoy spotting various bird species, including swans, ducks, and herons, which are commonly seen along the lake. If you're lucky, you might even catch a glimpse of a beaver or otter playing near the water's edge.

History buffs will appreciate the historical features scattered along the trail. In Geneva, you can visit landmarks like the Jet d'Eau fountain and the United Nations headquarters. As you move east, the town of Nyon boasts a Roman museum and ruins, giving insight into the region's ancient past. Lausanne offers cultural gems like the Olympic Museum and the medieval Lausanne Cathedral. Montreux, renowned for its annual jazz festival, is home to the Chillon Castle, a beautifully preserved medieval fortress that has inspired artists and writers for centuries.

The trail itself is divided into manageable sections, each with its unique charm and attractions. For example, the stretch from Geneva to Nyon is about 30 kilometers (18.6 miles) and takes around 7 to 8 hours to complete. This section is relatively flat and perfect for a leisurely day hike. The route from Lausanne to Montreux, approximately 30 kilometers (18.6 miles) as well, can take about 8 hours and offers breathtaking views of the lake, passing through vineyards and quaint villages. Each segment of the trail is well-serviced by public transportation, allowing hikers to easily start and stop their journey as they please.

The difficulty level of the Lake Geneva Trail is generally rated as easy to moderate. The well-maintained paths and gentle inclines make it suitable for families and casual hikers. However, the total distance can be challenging for those aiming to complete the entire trail in one go, so it's important to plan accordingly and pace yourself.

Pet owners will be pleased to know that dogs are welcome on the Lake Geneva Trail. However, regulations require that dogs be kept on a leash in certain areas, particularly in towns and near wildlife habitats to ensure the safety of both pets and local fauna. It's always a good idea to carry enough water for your dog and to be mindful of the weather, as some sections of the trail can be exposed to the sun.

Recommended Closest Accommodation

Geneva: (Hotel Central Geneva: Rue de la Rôtisserie 2, 1204 Geneva. This centrally located hotel offers comfortable rooms and easy access to the trailhead, providing a convenient starting point for your hike.)

(Hotel Longemalle: Place Longemalle 13, 1204 Geneva. Just steps from the lake, this elegant hotel offers excellent amenities and beautiful views.)

Nyon: (Base Nyon: Rue Jules Gachet 2, 1260 Nyon. A modern and stylish option located close to the train station and the lakeside trail.)

(Hotel Real: Place de Savoie 1, 1260 Nyon. Overlooking the lake, this hotel offers comfortable rooms and a great location near the trail.)

Recommended Closest Place to Eat

Geneva: (La Buvette des Bains: Quai du Mont-Blanc 30, 1201 Geneva. A popular spot by the lake offering Swiss dishes and a relaxed atmosphere.)

(Restaurant Edelweiss: Place de la Navigation 2, 1201 Geneva. Known for its traditional Swiss cuisine and charming setting.)

Nyon: (Le Café du Marché: Place du Marché 20, 1260 Nyon. A cozy eatery offering local specialties and friendly service.)

(Auberge de la Grenade: Rue de Rive 35, 1260 Nyon. A charming restaurant with a great menu featuring regional dishes.)

Logistics Upon Arrival

Parking and Cost: In Geneva, parking is available at several public garages such as Parking de Plainpalais, Rue de Carouge 7, 1205 Geneva, costing CHF 2 to CHF 4 per hour. Nyon offers parking at Parc de la Duche, Route de Saint-Cergue 6, 1260 Nyon, with rates around CHF 1.50 to CHF 2.50 per hour. In Lausanne, you can park at Parking Mon-Repos, Avenue du Tribunal-Fédéral 4, 1005 Lausanne, costing CHF 2 to CHF 3 per hour. Montreux provides parking at Parking du Marché-Forum, Rue du Marché, 1820 Montreux, with similar hourly rates.

Location (in relation to roads and towns)

The Lake Geneva Trail is easily accessible from major roads and towns. Geneva, located at the western tip of Lake Geneva, is well-connected by highways and public transport. From Geneva, you can follow the trail along the lakeshore to Nyon, approximately 30 kilometers away. Nyon itself is a picturesque town located along the main railway line and accessible via the A1 motorway. Continuing east, Lausanne is situated on the northern shore of Lake Geneva and is a major transport hub, easily accessible by road and rail. Montreux, further along the shore, can be reached via the A9 motorway or by train, making it an easy destination to include in your itinerary.

Directions

For directions to each segment of the Lake Geneva Trail, detailed addresses and GPS coordinates are useful. If starting in Geneva, you can begin at the iconic Jet d'Eau fountain located at Quai Gustave-Ador, 1207 Geneva. GPS coordinates: 46.2074° N, 6.1550° E. From here, the trail leads along the lakeside towards Nyon. To reach Nyon, set your destination to the Nyon Train Station at Place de la Gare 1, 1260 Nyon. GPS coordinates 46.3818° N, 6.2383° E. From Nyon, the trail continues towards Lausanne, where you can start near the Lausanne Train Station at Place de la Gare 5, 1003 Lausanne. GPS coordinates: 46.5170° N, 6.6296° E. Finally, for Montreux, you can begin at the Montreux Train Station located at Place de la Gare 3, 1820 Montreux. GPS coordinates: 46.4312° N, 6.9103° E.

Each of these starting points is conveniently located near public transport and parking facilities, making your arrival and departure straightforward.

Lauterbrunnen Valley Walk

The Lauterbrunnen Valley Walk begins in the heart of Lauterbrunnen village. This hike is suitable for most fitness levels, including families, and offers a relatively easy trek through some of the most stunning scenery in the Swiss Alps. The trail is well-marked, ensuring a hassle-free experience for all hikers.

Detailed Trail Descriptions

Starting at the Lauterbrunnen train station (GPS coordinates 46.5935° N, 7.9078° E), the trail kicks off with a gentle walk through the picturesque village. You'll soon encounter Staubbach Falls, a 300-meter-high waterfall that is one of the highest free-falling waterfalls in Europe. This early part of the trail is on paved paths, making it accessible and enjoyable.

From Staubbach Falls, the path continues towards Trümmelbach Falls, a distance of about 3 kilometers. The trail here is a mix of paved paths and gravel tracks, winding through lush meadows dotted with traditional Swiss chalets. Along this stretch, you'll pass by vibrant alpine roses, delicate edelweiss, and other wildflowers that add bursts of color to the landscape. Keep an eye out for historical barns and farmhouses that provide a glimpse into the valley's agricultural past.

Reaching Trümmelbach Falls, located at an altitude of 848 meters, you'll find a series of ten glacier-fed waterfalls hidden inside the mountain. Accessible via tunnels and platforms, this section involves some uphill walking and steps, making it moderately challenging. The thunderous roar and the sheer power of the water are truly awe-inspiring, and interpretive signs along the way offer insights into the falls' geology and hydrology.

The final stretch from Trümmelbach Falls to Stechelberg is about 4 kilometers of serene meadows and pastures. This part of the trail is on gravel paths and wooden bridges, offering a peaceful end to your hike. Wildlife such as marmots, chamois, and various bird species like golden eagles and alpine choughs can often be spotted in this area.

Trail Highlights Several features make the Lauterbrunnen Valley Walk exceptional. Staubbach Falls, visible from the village, is a dramatic start to your hike. The unique Trümmelbach Falls, with its powerful waterfalls inside the mountain, is a must-see. Along the trail, you'll traverse beautiful alpine meadows filled with wildflowers and have opportunities to observe local wildlife. Traditional Swiss farmhouses add a touch of history and culture to the experience.

Hike Specifications

The hike covers a total distance of 8 kilometers (5 miles) and typically takes around 3 to 4 hours to complete, depending on your pace and the number of stops you make. The trail has a gentle grade, with some steeper sections around Trümmelbach Falls, making it suitable for most hikers. The difficulty level is easy to moderate.

Regulations

Pets are welcome on the trail, but dogs should be kept on a leash, especially around livestock and wildlife areas. It's important to stay on marked paths to protect the delicate alpine environment. Be sure to carry out all trash and follow the Leave No Trace principles to help preserve the natural beauty of the area.

Accommodation Recommendations

For those looking to stay overnight, Hotel Staubbach offers stunning views of Staubbach Falls and comfortable rooms with modern amenities. Located on Hauptstrasse, 3822 Lauterbrunnen, it provides a convenient base for your hiking adventure.

Another great option is Camping Jungfrau, located at Weid 406, 3822 Lauterbrunnen. This campsite offers a range of accommodations from tents to cozy cabins, along with excellent facilities including a restaurant and a shop.

Dining Recommendations

After a day on the trail, enjoy a meal at the Hotel Oberland Restaurant, located at Fuhren, 3822 Lauterbrunnen. This restaurant offers traditional Swiss dishes and international favorites, focusing on locally sourced ingredients.

For a lighter meal or a snack, Airtime Café at Dorf, 3822 Lauterbrunnen, is a perfect choice. They serve sandwiches, pastries, and other light fare, ideal for a post-hike treat.

Logistics and Arrival

Parking in Lauterbrunnen Village is convenient, with several parking areas near the train station. The cost is approximately CHF 10-15 per day, and the parking locations are within walking distance of the trailhead.

To reach Lauterbrunnen by train, take the Berner Oberland Bahn (BOB) from Interlaken. The scenic ride takes about 20 minutes. If driving, follow signs for Lauterbrunnen from Interlaken. The drive is approximately 15 kilometers and takes around 20 minutes.

Hiking Guide Recommendation For those seeking a guided experience, Alpine Adventure Guides offers expert-led hikes in the

Lauterbrunnen Valley. You can contact them at info@alpineadventureguides.ch. Their knowledgeable guides provide valuable insights into the local environment, history, and geology, enhancing your hiking experience.

Appenzell Circular Trail

The Appenzell Circular Trail is a delightful hike that showcases the rustic charm of the Appenzell region in northeastern Switzerland. This circular route offers a blend of lush meadows, rolling hills, traditional Swiss villages, and panoramic mountain views. Along the way, hikers can expect to encounter a variety of flora and fauna, including alpine wildflowers, grazing cows, and perhaps even a shy ibex.

Trail Highlights

Highlights of the Appenzell Circular Trail include sweeping vistas of the Alpstein mountain range, picturesque Swiss chalets adorned with colorful flowers, and quaint villages where time seems to stand still. The trail also passes by historical landmarks such as ancient churches and traditional cheese dairies, offering insight into the region's rich cultural heritage.

Altitude, Length, and Difficulty Level

The trail typically starts and ends in the town of Appenzell and covers a distance of approximately 12 kilometers (7.5 miles). With a total elevation gain of around 400 meters (1,312 feet), the hike is considered moderate in difficulty, suitable for hikers of all skill levels.

Route Outline

The circular trail winds its way through the rolling hills and verdant pastures of the Appenzell countryside, passing through charming villages like Wasserauen, Schwellbrunn, and Gonten. Hikers can expect a mix of paved paths, gravel tracks, and narrow footpaths, with plenty of signposts along the way to guide their journey.

Regulations

Pets are generally allowed on the Appenzell Circular Trail but should be kept on a leash, especially in areas with livestock. Hikers are also encouraged to respect private property and adhere to local regulations regarding waste disposal and environmental protection.

Closest Accommodation: (Hotel Hecht Appenzell: Hauptgasse 9, 9050 Appenzell. This charming hotel is located in the heart of Appenzell's historic Old Town, offering comfortable rooms and easy access to the trailhead.) (**Guesthouse Krone**: Dorf 16, 9057 Wasserauen. Situated in the picturesque village of Wasserauen, this cozy guesthouse provides a peaceful retreat after a day of hiking.)

Closest Places to Eat: (Restaurant Alpenrose: Poststrasse 1, 9050 Appenzell. A popular dining spot known for its traditional Swiss cuisine and warm hospitality.) (**Gasthof Bären**: Dorf 39, 9057 Wasserauen. This rustic inn serves hearty regional dishes and boasts a sunny terrace with stunning mountain views.)

Logistics Upon Arrival Parking is available in Appenzell at various public lots, with hourly rates typically ranging from CHF 1 to CHF

2.50. The trailhead is easily accessible from the town center, either on foot or by public transport. Appenzell is well-connected by road and rail, making it a convenient starting point for your hike.

Location

Appenzell is located in the canton of Appenzell Innerrhoden in northeastern Switzerland. It is accessible by road via the A1 motorway and by train from major cities like Zurich and St. Gallen.

Directions

By Car: From Zurich, take the A1 motorway east towards St. Gallen. Take exit 80-Appenzell toward Schwende/Appenzell. Follow signs for Appenzell and park in one of the public lots in the town center.

By Train: Direct trains run from Zurich to Appenzell, with a travel time of approximately 1.5 hours. The trailhead is a short walk from the Appenzell train station.

Recommended Hiking Guide Company

Appenzellerland Tourismus AI. They offer knowledgeable guides who can lead you on customized tours tailored to your interests and fitness level.

Oeschinensee Panorama Trail

The Oeschinensee Panorama Trail offers a breathtaking journey through the stunning landscapes of the Bernese Oberland. This scenic hike showcases the beauty of the Swiss Alps, with panoramic views of snow-capped peaks, crystal-clear mountain lakes, and lush alpine meadows. Hikers can expect to encounter a diverse range of flora and fauna, including alpine flowers, marmots, and perhaps even a golden eagle soaring overhead.

Trail Highlights

Highlights of the Oeschinensee Panorama Trail include the iconic Oeschinensee Lake, one of Switzerland's most picturesque alpine lakes, and the towering peaks of the Bluemlisalp massif. The trail also passes by traditional mountain huts and charming chalets, where hikers can stop for a refreshing drink or a taste of local Swiss cuisine.

Altitude, Length, and Difficulty Level

The trail typically starts at the Oeschinen Lake gondola station and covers a distance of approximately 5 kilometers (3.1 miles) one way, with a total elevation gain of around 200 meters (656 feet). The hike is considered moderate in difficulty, with well-marked paths and gentle gradients suitable for hikers of all abilities.

Route Outline

The Oeschinensee Panorama Trail follows a loop route around the shores of Oeschinen Lake, offering stunning views of the surrounding mountains and valleys. Hikers can choose to start from either the gondola station or the lakeside parking area, with the option to extend the hike by exploring additional trails in the area.

Regulations

Pets are generally allowed on the Oeschinensee Panorama Trail but should be kept on a leash, especially in areas with wildlife or grazing livestock. Hikers are also reminded to respect the natural environment and follow Leave No Trace principles by packing out any waste and staying on designated trails.

Closest Accommodation: (Berghotel Oeschinensee: Kandersteg, 3718 Kandersteg. Situated directly on the shores of Oeschinen Lake, this mountain hotel offers cozy rooms and stunning views of the surrounding peaks.) (**Hotel Alpenblick Kandersteg**: Usser Klus 19, 3718 Kandersteg. Located in the charming village of Kandersteg, this family-run hotel provides comfortable accommodation and easy access to the trailhead.)

Closest Places to Eat: (Restaurant Oeschinensee: Oeschinensee, 3718 Kandersteg. This lakeside restaurant serves delicious Swiss specialties and offers outdoor seating with panoramic views of the lake and mountains.) (**Hotel Alpenblick Restaurant**: Usser Klus 19, 3718 Kandersteg. The hotel's restaurant serves a variety of hearty mountain dishes and is a popular spot for hikers and visitors alike.)

Logistics Upon Arrival

Parking is available at the Oeschinen Lake parking area, with hourly rates typically ranging from CHF 1 to CHF 2.50. The gondola station is located nearby, providing easy access to the trailhead. Kandersteg is the nearest town and is accessible by road and rail from major cities like Bern and Zurich.

Location

The Oeschinensee Panorama Trail is located near the village of Kandersteg in the Bernese Oberland region of Switzerland. Kandersteg is easily accessible by road via the A6 motorway and by train from major cities like Bern and Zurich.

Directions

By Car: From Bern or Zurich, take the A6 motorway to the Kandersteg exit. Follow signs for Kandersteg and continue to the Oeschinen Lake parking area.

By Train: Direct trains run from Bern or Zurich to Kandersteg, with a travel time of approximately 1.5 to 2 hours. From Kandersteg, take the gondola or hike to the Oeschinen Lake trailhead.

Recommended Hiking Guide Company: **Alpine Hikers Switzerland**. They offer experienced guides who can lead you on personalized tours tailored to your interests and fitness level.

Grindelwald First Cliff Walk

The Grindelwald First Cliff Walk is an exhilarating hike that offers jaw-dropping views of the Eiger, Monch, and Jungfrau peaks. This unique trail features a series of suspension bridges and viewing platforms, allowing hikers to experience the thrill of walking above the abyss while soaking in the beauty of the Swiss Alps. Highlights of the Grindelwald First Cliff Walk include the stunning vistas of the surrounding mountains and glaciers, the adrenaline rush of crossing the suspension bridges, and the opportunity to learn about the region's geology and wildlife at interpretive stations along the way.

Altitude, Length, and Difficulty Level

The trail typically starts at the First gondola station and covers a distance of approximately 2 kilometers (1.2 miles) round trip, with minimal elevation gain. The hike is considered easy to moderate in difficulty, with well-maintained paths and sturdy bridges suitable for hikers of all ages and abilities.

Route Outline

The Grindelwald First Cliff Walk follows a loop route from the First gondola station, crossing two suspension bridges and passing several viewing platforms along the way. Hikers can choose to start from either the gondola station or the nearby mountain restaurant, with the option to extend the hike by exploring additional trails in the area.

Regulations

Pets are generally not allowed on the Grindelwald First Cliff Walk due to safety reasons and the fragile nature of the infrastructure. Hikers are reminded to stay on designated paths and respect any posted signs or guidelines to ensure a safe and enjoyable experience for themselves and others.

Closest Accommodation

Hotel Belvedere Grindelwald: Dorfstrasse 53, 3818 Grindelwald. Situated in Grindelwald's town center, this hotel offers comfortable rooms and stunning views of the surrounding mountains, providing a convenient base for exploring the area. 2. **Hotel Kirchbühl Grindelwald**: Obere Gletscherstrasse 3, 3818 Grindelwald. Nestled amidst the alpine scenery, this charming hotel offers cozy accommodation and easy access to the First gondola station.

Closest Places to Eat: (Restaurant First: Bergrestaurant First, 3818 Grindelwald. Located near the First gondola station, this restaurant offers a variety of Swiss and international dishes, with indoor and outdoor seating options.) (**Berggasthaus Bort**: Bort, 3818 Grindelwald. Situated midway along the trail, this mountain restaurant serves hearty alpine cuisine and boasts panoramic views of the surrounding peaks.)

Logistics Upon Arrival

Parking is available at the Grindelwald First gondola station, with hourly rates typically ranging from CHF 1.50 to CHF 3. The gondola station is easily accessible from Grindelwald's town center, either on foot or by public transport. Grindelwald is well-connected by road and rail, making it a convenient starting point for your hike.

Location

The Grindelwald First Cliff Walk is located near the town of Grindelwald in the Bernese Oberland region of Switzerland.

Grindelwald is accessible by road via the A8 motorway and by train from major cities like Bern and Zurich.

Directions

By Car: From Bern or Zurich, take the A8 motorway to the Grindelwald exit. Follow signs for Grindelwald and continue to the First gondola station.

By Train: Direct trains run from Bern or Zurich to Grindelwald, with a travel time of approximately 2 to 2.5 hours. From Grindelwald's train station, take the local bus or walk to the First Gondola station.

Recommended Hiking Guide Company: Grindelwald Sports. They offer experienced guides who can lead you on thrilling adventures in the Swiss Alps, including the Grindelwald First Cliff Walk.

Männlichen Royal Walk

The Männlichen Royal Walk is a regal hike that offers majestic views of the Jungfrau region's most iconic peaks. This stroll follows a scenic ridge between the Männlichen and Kleine Scheidegg mountains, offering panoramic vistas of the Eiger, Monch, and Jungfrau summits. Highlights of the Männlichen Royal Walk include the stunning alpine scenery, the opportunity to spot ibex and marmots along the way, and the chance to learn about the region's geology and history at interpretive stations along the route.

Altitude, Length, and Difficulty Level

The trail typically starts at the Männlichen gondola station and covers a distance of approximately 2.5 kilometers (1.5 miles) one way, with minimal elevation gain. The hike is considered easy, with well-marked paths and gentle gradients suitable for hikers of all ages and fitness levels.

Route Outline

The Männlichen Royal Walk follows a gentle ridge between the Männlichen and Kleine Scheidegg mountains, offering stunning views of the surrounding peaks and valleys. Hikers can choose to start from either the Männlichen gondola station or the Kleine Scheidegg railway station, with the option to extend the hike by exploring additional trails in the area.

Regulations

Pets are generally allowed on the Männlichen Royal Walk but should be kept on a leash, especially in areas with wildlife or grazing livestock. Hikers are reminded to stay on designated paths and respect any posted signs or guidelines to ensure a safe and enjoyable experience for themselves and others.

Closest Accommodation: (Hotel Bellevue des Alpes: 3818 Grindelwald. Situated at Kleine Scheidegg, this historic hotel offers comfortable rooms and stunning views of the Eiger, Monch, and Jungfrau peaks.). (**Berghotel Männlichen**: 3823 Wengen. Located at the Männlichen summit, this mountain hotel provides cozy accommodation and easy access to the trailhead.)

Closest Places to Eat: (Restaurant Panorama: Kleine Scheidegg, 3823 Wengen. This mountain restaurant serves a variety of Swiss and international dishes, with panoramic views of the surrounding peaks.) **(Restaurant Männlichen**: Männlichen, 3823 Wengen. Situated at the Männlichen gondola station, this restaurant offers alpine cuisine and outdoor seating with breathtaking views of the Jungfrau region.)

Logistics Upon Arrival

Parking is available at the Grindelwald or Lauterbrunnen train stations, with hourly rates typically ranging from CHF 1.50 to CHF 3. The Männlichen gondola station is easily accessible from both stations, either by train or by bus. Grindelwald and Lauterbrunnen are well-connected by road and rail, making them convenient starting points for your hike.

Location

The Männlichen Royal Walk is located in the Jungfrau region of the Bernese Oberland, near the towns of Grindelwald and Lauterbrunnen. Grindelwald and Lauterbrunnen are accessible by road via the A8 motorway and by train from major cities like Bern and Zurich.

Directions By Car: From Bern or Zurich, take the A8 motorway to Grindelwald or Lauterbrunnen. Follow signs for the Männlichen gondola station or Kleine Scheidegg railway station.

By Train: Direct trains run from Bern or Zurich to Grindelwald or Lauterbrunnen, with a travel time of approximately 2 to 2.5 hours. From Grindelwald or Lauterbrunnen's train station, take the local bus or train to the Männlichen gondola station or Kleine Scheidegg railway station.

Muggestutz Fairy Tale Trail

The Muggestutz Fairy Tale Trail is a delightful family-friendly hike in the Hasliberg region, designed to captivate both young and old with its whimsical charm. Spanning 5.5 kilometers, this easy trail ascends to an altitude of 1,500 meters, taking about two and a half hours to complete.

The trail tells the enchanting story of Muggestutz, the oldest dwarf in the Hasli region. Along the way, hikers will find interactive stations where children can play, explore, and learn about the fairy tale. The route is surrounded by lush meadows, vibrant wildflowers, and dense forests that provide a habitat for various wildlife such as deer, marmots, and numerous bird species. Additionally, hikers might encounter historical alpine huts and traditional Swiss farming practices still in use today.

For accommodations, the Hotel Gletscherblick at Oberer Gletscher 1, 3860 Meiringen, offers comfortable rooms and beautiful views. Another option is the Hotel Reuti, located at Engi 485, 6086 Hasliberg, known for its family-friendly amenities. For dining, try Restaurant Wasserwendi, located at Twing 365, 6084 Hasliberg Wasserwendi, for traditional Swiss cuisine. Alternatively, Restaurant Bären, at 6085 Hasliberg Goldern, offers local specialties in a cozy atmosphere.

Parking is available at the Hasliberg Reuti gondola station, costing around CHF 5 per day. The trailhead is accessible via a short gondola ride from Meiringen. By car, drive to Meiringen, then follow signs to Hasliberg Reuti. Public transport options include taking a train to Meiringen, and then a bus to Hasliberg Reuti.

For guided tours, the Haslital Tourism office offers knowledgeable guides who can enhance the experience with stories and local insights.

Stoos Ridge Hike

The Stoos Ridge Hike is a breathtaking trail offering panoramic views of Lake Lucerne and the surrounding Alps. Stretching 10 kilometers, the trail reaches an altitude of 1,936 meters and is considered moderate in difficulty, taking about four hours to complete.

Starting in the village of Stoos, the hike follows a ridge with dramatic drops on either side, providing spectacular vistas throughout. Hikers will traverse alpine meadows, encounter hardy mountain flora such as edelweiss and alpine roses, and may spot ibex and chamois. The trail also passes historical sites like old shepherd huts and offers insights into the region's alpine farming traditions.

For a comfortable stay, the Seminar- und Wellnesshotel Stoos at Ringstrasse 10, 6433 Stoos, provides excellent amenities and stunning views. Alternatively, the Gasthaus Balmberg at Balmberg 70, 4584 Lüterkofen-Ichertswil, offers cozy rooms and local hospitality. Dining options include Restaurant Klingenstock, situated at Stoosplatz 1, 6433 Stoos, known for its hearty Swiss dishes. Another choice is the

Gipfelrestaurant Fronalpstock, located at the summit station of the Fronalpstock chairlift.

Parking is available at the Stoos funicular lower station in Schlattli, costing about CHF 7 per day. The hike starts from the top of the funicular in Stoos. By car, drive to Schwyz, then follow signs to the Stoosbahn funicular. Public transport options include taking a train to Schwyz, then a bus to the funicular station in Schlattli.

For a guided experience, the Stoos-Muotathal Tourism office offers professional guides who provide detailed information about the trail and the surrounding area.

Gruyères Cheese Trail

The Gruyères Cheese Trail combines stunning scenery with a culinary journey through the Swiss countryside. This 12-kilometer trail, which takes about four hours to hike, reaches an altitude of 1,180 meters and is suitable for hikers of all levels.

Starting in the picturesque town of Gruyères, the trail winds through lush pastures and forests, offering views of the medieval Gruyères Castle and the Moléson Peak. Along the way, hikers can see cows grazing and visit local dairies to learn about the traditional methods of cheese-making. The trail is rich in flora, including wildflowers and alpine plants, and fauna such as deer and various bird species.

For accommodations, consider staying at the Hotel de Ville, located at Rue du Bourg 29, 1663 Gruyères, which offers historic charm and comfortable rooms. Another excellent choice is the Hostellerie Saint-Georges, at Rue du Bourg 22, 1663 Gruyères, known for its beautiful setting and friendly service. Dining options include Le Chalet de Gruyères at Rue du Bourg 56, 1663 Gruyères, famous for its fondue and local dishes. Another recommended restaurant is La Maison du Gruyère at Place de la Gare 3, 1663 Pringy-Gruyères, where you can taste authentic Gruyères cheese.

Parking is available in the Gruyères village parking lot, costing about CHF 5 per day. The trailhead is easily accessible from the village center. By car, drive to Gruyères and follow signs to the village parking. Public transport options include taking a train to Gruyères station.

For a guided tour, the Gruyères Tourism office offers knowledgeable guides who can provide insights into the region's history, culture, and cheese-making traditions.

Rigi Panorama Trail

The Rigi Panorama Trail offers breathtaking views of Lake Lucerne and the surrounding Swiss Alps. This 7-kilometer trail, which takes about three hours to hike, reaches an altitude of 1,798 meters and is classified as easy, making it suitable for all fitness levels.

The trail begins at the Rigi Kaltbad station and winds its way through alpine meadows and forests. Hikers will enjoy stunning panoramic views, including sights of Mount Pilatus and the distant Jura Mountains. The trail features a variety of alpine flora, such as gentians and mountain pines, and wildlife including marmots and golden eagles.

Historical highlights include the Rigi Kaltbad Mineral Baths, a popular spa destination since the 16th century.

For accommodations, the Hotel Rigi Kaltbad at 6356 Rigi Kaltbad offers modern amenities and spectacular views. Another option is the Hotel Rigi First at Firstweg 4, 6356 Rigi Kaltbad, which provides comfortable rooms and excellent service. Dining options include the Panorama Restaurant at 6356 Rigi Kaltbad, known for its local cuisine and stunning views. Alternatively, the Restaurant Bärenstube, located at Rigi Kaltbad, offers traditional Swiss dishes in a cozy setting.

Parking is available at the Weggis cable car station, costing about CHF 10 per day. The trailhead is accessible via the Rigi Kaltbad cable car. By car, drive to Weggis and follow signs to the cable car station. Public transport options include taking a train to Lucerne, then a boat to Weggis, followed by the cable car to Rigi Kaltbad.

For guided hikes, the Rigi Tourism office offers experienced guides who can enrich your hike with local knowledge and fascinating stories about the region.

Aare Gorge Trail

The Aare Gorge Trail offers a dramatic and awe-inspiring hike through a natural rock formation carved by the Aare River over thousands of years. This 1.4-kilometer trail is relatively easy and suitable for all ages, with a gentle elevation reaching 710 meters. The hike typically takes about an hour to complete.

The trail begins at the west entrance in Meiringen and continues through the gorge, featuring narrow pathways and tunnels that bring hikers close to the roaring river below. The walls of the gorge tower up to 200 meters high, creating an impressive natural spectacle. Along the way, you'll encounter lush vegetation clinging to the rock faces, including mosses, ferns, and alpine flowers. Wildlife such as trout can be seen in the crystal-clear waters, and if you're lucky, you might spot birds of prey soaring above.

For accommodations, consider the Hotel Victoria at Bahnhofplatz 9, 3860 Meiringen, offering stylish rooms and excellent service. Another good choice is the Parkhotel du Sauvage at Bahnhofstrasse 30, 3860 Meiringen, known for its historic charm and comfortable amenities. For dining, try Restaurant Baertschi, located at Bahnhofplatz 11, 3860 Meiringen, which offers traditional Swiss cuisine. Alternatively, enjoy a meal at Hotel Restaurant Alpbach at Kirchgasse 17, 3860 Meiringen, known for its fine dining and local specialties.

Parking is available at the Aare Gorge west entrance for about CHF 5 per day. The trailhead is easy to reach from the center of Meiringen. By car, follow signs to Meiringen and then to the Aare Gorge west entrance. Public transport options include taking a train to Meiringen, followed by a short walk to the entrance.

For guided tours, the Haslital Tourism office provides knowledgeable guides who can offer insights into the geological and historical aspects of the gorge.

Seebenalp Panorama Trail

The Seebenalp Panorama Trail is a scenic hike that offers breathtaking views of Lake Walen and the surrounding Churfirsten peaks. This 8-kilometer trail is moderately difficult, with an altitude of 1,600 meters, and takes around three hours to complete.

Starting at the Flumserberg Tannenboden, the trail meanders through alpine meadows and dense forests, providing stunning panoramic vistas along the way. The route is dotted with colorful wildflowers such as gentians and edelweiss in the summer, and you might spot marmots and chamois. Historical features include old mountain huts and remnants of ancient stone walls.

For accommodations, the Hotel Cristal Flumserberg at Tannenbodenalp, 8898 Flumserberg, offers cozy rooms and excellent views. Another option is the Hotel Siesta, located at Tannenboden, 8898 Flumserberg, known for its friendly service and comfortable amenities. Dining options include the Restaurant Sennästube at Tannenbodenalp, 8898 Flumserberg, which serves delicious Swiss dishes. Another recommendation is the Molseralp Restaurant, at Tannenboden, 8898 Flumserberg, known for its local specialties.

Parking is available at the Flumserberg Tannenboden for about CHF 10 per day. The trailhead is accessible from Tannenbodenalp. By car, drive to Flumserberg and follow signs to Tannenbodenalp. Public transport options include taking a train to Unterterzen, and then a bus to Flumserberg Tannenboden.

For a guided experience, the Flumserberg Tourism office offers professional guides who can provide in-depth information about the trail and its natural features.

Trummelbach Falls Loop Trail

The Trummelbach Falls Loop Trail offers a thrilling hike through a series of ten glacier-fed waterfalls inside a mountain in the Lauterbrunnen Valley. This 2-kilometer trail is easy and accessible, with an altitude of 980 meters and taking about one hour to complete.

The trail begins at the Trummelbach Falls entrance and follows a loop that includes elevators and walkways leading to the waterfalls. The falls, fed by the melting snow from the Eiger, Mönch, and Jungfrau mountains, thunder through the narrow crevices with immense force. The trail also features lush vegetation, with ferns and mosses thriving in the moist environment. Wildlife in the area includes alpine birds and occasionally mountain goats.

For accommodations, the Hotel Silberhorn at Bir Zuben 465, 3822 Lauterbrunnen, offers comfortable rooms and excellent service. Another option is the Hotel Staubbach at Hauptstrasse, 3822 Lauterbrunnen, known for its cozy atmosphere and friendly staff. Dining options include the Hotel Oberland Restaurant at Fuhren, 3822 Lauterbrunnen, which serves traditional Swiss cuisine. Another recommendation is the Airtime Cafe, at Dorf 3822, Lauterbrunnen, known for its fresh pastries and coffee.

Parking is available at the Trummelbach Falls entrance for about CHF 5 per day. The trailhead is located at the falls entrance, easily accessible from Lauterbrunnen. By car, drive to Lauterbrunnen and follow signs to the Trummelbach Falls. Public transport options include taking a train to Lauterbrunnen, and then a bus to the falls.

For guided tours, the Lauterbrunnen Tourism office offers knowledgeable guides who can enhance your visit with detailed information about the falls and their geological significance.

Interlaken Panorama Trail

The Interlaken Panorama Trail provides stunning views of the lakes Thun and Brienz, as well as the surrounding mountains. This 6-kilometer trail is moderately difficult, with an altitude of 1,322 meters, and takes about two and a half hours to complete.

Starting from the Harder Kulm, the trail offers breathtaking panoramic views right from the start. The path winds through alpine meadows and forests, featuring diverse flora such as alpine roses and mountain pines. Wildlife sightings may include ibex and eagles. Historical features along the trail include old farming terraces and traditional wooden chalets.

For accommodations, consider staying at the Hotel Interlaken at Höheweg 74, 3800 Interlaken, which offers historic charm and modern amenities. Another excellent choice is the Hotel Beausite, located at

Seestrasse 16, 3800 Interlaken, known for its friendly service and comfortable rooms. Dining options include Restaurant Taverne at Höheweg 37, 3800 Interlaken, which serves Swiss and international dishes. Alternatively, the Harder Kulm Panorama Restaurant at Harder Kulm, 3800 Interlaken, offers delicious food with a view.

Parking is available at the Harderbahn station for about CHF 10 per day. The trailhead is accessible from the Harder Kulm, which can be reached by a funicular from Interlaken. By car, drive to Interlaken and follow signs to the Harderbahn station. Public transport options include taking a train to Interlaken Ost and then walking to the funicular station.

For guided hikes, the Interlaken Tourism office offers experienced guides who can provide fascinating insights into the natural and cultural history of the area.

Schynige Platte Loop Trail

The Schynige Platte Loop Trail is a scenic gem in the Bernese Oberland, offering panoramic views of the Eiger, Mönch, and Jungfrau peaks. This 6.5-kilometer trail, with an altitude of 2,076 meters, is moderately difficult and takes around three hours to complete.

Starting from the Schynige Platte railway station, the trail winds through alpine meadows adorned with wildflowers like gentians, alpine roses, and edelweiss. The route offers glimpses of diverse wildlife, including marmots, chamois, and golden eagles. The historical Schynige Platte Railway, dating back to 1893, adds a nostalgic touch to the hike, as does the Alpine Garden, showcasing over 600 species of alpine plants.

For accommodations, consider the Hotel Berghaus at Schynige Platte, 3812 Wilderswil, offering cozy rooms and breathtaking views. Another excellent option is the Hotel Alpenblick at Oberdorfstrasse 3, 3812 Wilderswil, known for its charming ambiance and comfortable amenities. For dining, the Panorama Restaurant at Schynige Platte serves hearty Swiss cuisine with a view, located at the top station of the Schynige Platte Railway. Alternatively, enjoy a meal at the Hotel Restaurant Heimat in Wilderswil, at Kirchgasse 72, offering traditional dishes in a rustic setting.

Parking is available at the Wilderswil railway station for about CHF 5 per day. The trailhead is accessible via the Schynige Platte Railway from Wilderswil. By car, drive to Wilderswil and follow signs to the railway station. Public transport options include taking a train to Wilderswil, and then transferring to the Schynige Platte Railway.

For guided hikes, the Jungfrau Region Tourism office offers knowledgeable guides who can enrich your experience with insights into the natural and historical highlights of the area.

Zurich Uetliberg Panorama Trail

The Zurich Uetliberg Panorama Trail is a popular escape from the city, offering stunning views of Zurich, Lake Zurich, and the Alps. This 7-kilometer trail, at an altitude of 870 meters, is easy and takes about two and a half hours to complete.

Starting at the Uetliberg station, the trail follows a scenic route along the ridge, passing through dense forests and open meadows. The path is lined with beech and oak trees, and in spring, the ground is carpeted with wildflowers. Wildlife such as foxes and various bird species can often be spotted. The Uetliberg Tower provides an excellent vantage point to appreciate the panoramic views.

For accommodations, the Uto Kulm Hotel at Uetliberg 451, 8143 Zurich, offers modern rooms and a serene atmosphere. Another option is the Hotel Ascot at Tessinerplatz 9, 8002 Zurich, known for its elegant decor and convenient location. For dining, the Uto Kulm Restaurant at Uetliberg 451 serves delicious Swiss cuisine with a view. Alternatively, the Restaurant Gmuetliberg at Uetliberg 15 offers traditional dishes in a cozy setting.

Parking is available at the Uitikon-Waldegg station, with a fee of around CHF 10 per day. The trailhead is accessible via a short train ride on the Sihltalbahn to Uetliberg. By car, drive to Uitikon-Waldegg and park at the station. Public transport options include taking a train to Zurich HB, then the Sihltalbahn to Uetliberg.

For a guided hike, the Zurich Tourism office provides experienced guides who can offer detailed information about the trail and the surrounding area.

Lake Thun Promenade

The Lake Thun Promenade offers a leisurely hike along the shores of Lake Thun, with stunning views of the surrounding mountains and charming lakeside villages. This 8-kilometer trail is easy and flat, taking about two hours to complete, with an altitude of around 558 meters.

Starting from Thun, the trail follows the lakeshore to the village of Hilterfingen. The route passes through beautiful parks and gardens, with an abundance of flora such as chestnut trees and roses. Along the way, hikers can enjoy views of historical castles like Schloss Thun and Schloss Hünegg. Waterfowl, such as swans and ducks, are commonly seen on the lake, adding to the serene atmosphere.

For accommodations, the Hotel Seepark at Seestrasse 47, 3602 Thun, offers luxurious rooms and lakeside views. Another option is the Hotel Bellevue au Lac at Staatsstrasse 1, 3652 Hilterfingen, known for its elegant ambiance and excellent service. For dining, try the Restaurant Chartreuse at Staatsstrasse 142, 3626 Hünibach, offering fine dining with a view. Alternatively, the Restaurant Dampfschiff at Freienhofgasse 10, 3600 Thun, serves traditional Swiss cuisine in a picturesque setting.

Parking is available at the Thun railway station, with a fee of around CHF 5 per day. The trailhead is easily accessible from the center of Thun. By car, drive to Thun and follow signs to the railway station. Public transport options include taking a train to Thun station.

For guided walks, the Thun Tourism office offers knowledgeable guides who can provide insights into the history and natural beauty of the area.

Rütli Meadow Trail

The Rütli Meadow Trail is a historic hike that leads to the birthplace of Switzerland, offering scenic views of Lake Lucerne and the surrounding mountains. This 5-kilometer trail, with an altitude of 500 meters, is easy and takes about one and a half hours to complete.

Starting from the Rütli boat dock, the trail winds through meadows and forests, passing by the famous Rütli Meadow where the Swiss Confederation was founded in 1291. The area is rich in flora, with wildflowers and old-growth trees, and fauna such as deer and various bird species. Historical markers along the trail recount the significant events that took place here.

For accommodations, consider the Hotel Seeburg at Seeburgstrasse 53-61, 6006 Lucerne, offering lakeside views and modern amenities. Another excellent choice is the Seehotel Hermitage at Seeburgstrasse 72, 6006 Lucerne, known for its serene location and comfortable rooms. For dining, the Restaurant Rütlihaus at Rütliwiese, 6452 Seelisberg, serves traditional Swiss dishes. Alternatively, the Restaurant Bahnhofli at Seelisberg, 6377 Seelisberg, offers local cuisine in a cozy setting.

Parking is available at the Seelisberg station, costing about CHF 5 per day. The trailhead is accessible by a boat ride from Brunnen or Lucerne to the Rütli dock. By car, drive to Seelisberg and park at the station. Public transport options include taking a train to Brunnen, and then a boat to Rütli. For guided tours, the Lucerne Tourism office provides experienced guides who can offer detailed historical context and enrich the hiking experience.

Aletsch Promenade

The Aletsch Promenade is a breathtaking trail that offers stunning views of the Aletsch Glacier, the largest glacier in the Alps. This 12-kilometer trail, with an altitude of around 2,200 meters, is moderately difficult and typically takes about four hours to complete.

Starting at the Bettmerhorn cable car station, the trail meanders along the ridgeline, offering panoramic views of the Aletsch Glacier and the surrounding peaks. The path is well-maintained and winds through alpine meadows and dense forests. The region is rich in flora, with vibrant wildflowers such as edelweiss and gentians, and ancient Arolla pines. Wildlife sightings may include ibex, marmots, and golden eagles soaring high above. Historical features include the charming alpine village of Bettmeralp, where traditional Swiss chalets and ancient barns dot the landscape.

For accommodations, consider the Hotel Waldhaus at Postfach 155, 3992 Bettmeralp, which offers comfortable rooms and stunning views. Another excellent choice is the Hotel Alpfrieden at Postfach 10, 3992 Bettmeralp, known for its warm hospitality and cozy ambiance. For dining, the Restaurant Bettmerhof at Hotel Bettmerhof, 3992 Bettmeralp, offers delicious Swiss cuisine and local specialties. Alternatively, the Panorama Restaurant Bettmerhorn at Bettmerhorn cable car station serves hearty meals with a view of the glacier.

Parking is available at the Betten Talstation for around CHF 8 per day. From there, take the cable car up to Bettmeralp and then the Bettmerhorn cable car to the trailhead. By car, drive to Betten and follow signs to the cable car station. Public transport options include taking a train to Betten Talstation and then the cable car up to Bettmeralp.

For guided hikes, the Aletsch Arena Tourism office offers knowledgeable guides who can provide insights into the geology, flora, and fauna of the area, enhancing the overall hiking experience.

Gelmersee Lake Trail

The Gelmersee Lake Trail is a thrilling hike that leads to the stunning Gelmersee Lake, nestled in the rugged Bernese Alps. This 6-kilometer trail, with an altitude of 1,850 meters, is moderately difficult and takes about three hours to complete.

Starting at the Gelmerbahn funicular station, the trail ascends steeply to the Gelmersee Lake, one of the most picturesque alpine lakes in Switzerland. The route offers spectacular views of the surrounding peaks and valleys. The path is surrounded by lush alpine meadows, vibrant wildflowers such as alpine asters and mountain daisies, and dense forests. Wildlife sightings might include chamois, marmots, and a variety of alpine birds. The highlight of this hike is Gelmersee Lake, with its crystal-clear turquoise waters reflecting the surrounding mountains.

For accommodations, the Hotel Grimsel Hospiz at Grimselpass, 3864 Guttannen, offers historic charm and comfortable rooms. Another excellent option is the Hotel Handeck at Handeck, 3864 Guttannen, known for its cozy ambiance and beautiful surroundings. For dining, the

Restaurant Grimsel Hospiz at Grimselpass, 3864 Guttannen, serves traditional Swiss cuisine with stunning views. Alternatively, the Restaurant Handeck at Handeck, 3864 Guttannen, offers local dishes in a rustic setting.

Parking is available at the Gelmerbahn funicular station for around CHF 10 per day. The trailhead is accessible via the Gelmerbahn funicular, which takes you up to the starting point of the hike. By car, drive to Guttannen and follow signs to the Gelmerbahn funicular station. Public transport options include taking a train to Meiringen, then a bus to Handegg, and finally the Gelmerbahn funicular.

For guided hikes, the Grimselwelt Tourism office provides experienced guides who can offer detailed information about the natural and historical aspects of the trail, making your hike both informative and enjoyable.

Chapter 3

Moderate Trails (For Hikers with Some Experience)

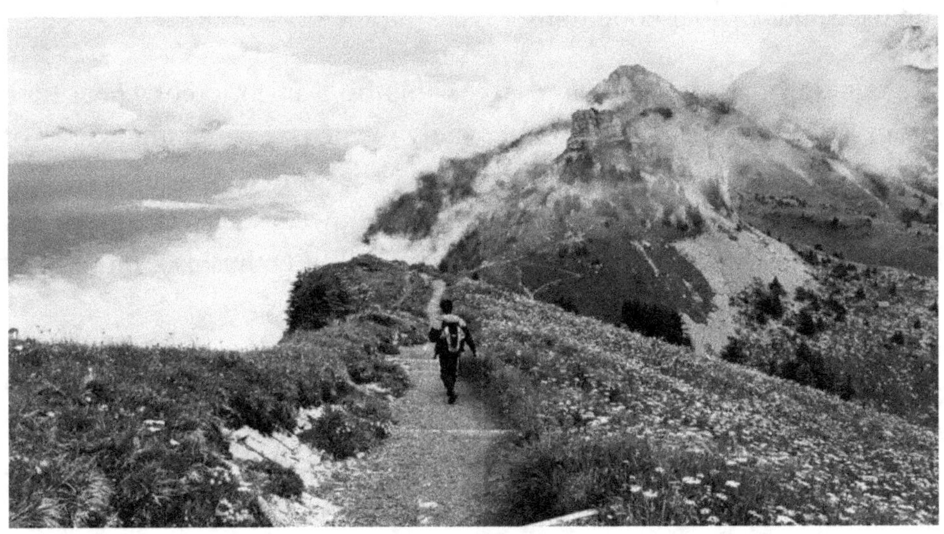

Each of these trails offers a unique glimpse into Switzerland's natural beauty, blending breathtaking landscapes with rich biodiversity and fascinating history. Whether you're seeking a stroll or a more challenging trek, these routes promise an unforgettable hiking adventure.

Schynige Platte to First Trail

The Schynige Platte to First Trail offers hikers a mesmerizing journey through Switzerland's Bernese Oberland, renowned for its sweeping views of the Alps, verdant meadows, and diverse flora and fauna. This trail stretches approximately 16 kilometers (10 miles) with an altitude range from 1,967 meters (6,453 feet) at Schynige Platte to 2,168 meters (7,113 feet) at First, posing a moderate to challenging level of difficulty. Typically, this hike can take around 6-7 hours to complete, depending on pace and weather conditions.

Beginning at Schynige Platte, accessible by a historic cogwheel train from Wilderswil, hikers are immediately greeted by panoramic views of the Eiger, Mönch, and Jungfrau peaks. The trail winds through lush meadows adorned with a variety of alpine flowers such as gentians and edelweiss during the summer months. Wildlife enthusiasts might spot marmots, chamois, and golden eagles soaring above.

As the trail progresses towards Faulhorn, one of the highest points on the route, the path becomes rockier, demanding careful footing. The historic Faulhorn Mountain Hotel, perched at 2,681 meters (8,796 feet), offers a charming rest stop with breathtaking vistas. Continuing towards First, the trail descends slightly, revealing serene alpine lakes and culminating in a dramatic ridge walk before reaching the First cable car station.

For accommodation, consider staying at the Hotel Schynige Platte, located at Schynige Platte, 3812 Wilderswil, or the Mountain Hostel Grindelwald, situated at Terrassenweg 104, 3818 Grindelwald. Both offer cozy lodgings with easy access to the trail.

Dining options include the Berghaus Männdlenen, located on the trail itself, providing hearty meals with spectacular views. Alternatively,

Restaurant Schreckfeld at First offers traditional Swiss cuisine with a panoramic terrace.

Parking is available at Wilderswil Train Station, costing around CHF 5 per day, where the cogwheel train to Schynige Platte departs. GPS coordinates for the station are 46.6642° N, 7.8666° E.

To reach the trailhead, take the train from Interlaken Ost to Wilderswil, then transfer to the cogwheel train to Schynige Platte. For a guided experience, Alpinehikers (Address: Grindelwaldstrasse 19, 3818 Grindelwald) offers expert-led hikes along this scenic route.

Muottas Muragl Panorama Trail

The Muottas Muragl Panorama Trail in the Engadin Valley offers stunning views of the Upper Engadin lakes and peaks. This 6.5-kilometer (4 miles) trail starts at an altitude of 2,454 meters (8,051 feet) and is relatively easy, making it suitable for most hikers. It typically takes about 2-3 hours to complete.

Starting from the Muottas Muragl funicular station, the trail follows a well-marked path offering panoramic views of the Piz Bernina massif and the Engadin valley below. The trail is adorned with alpine flora such as arnica and alpine roses. Red deer and ibex are often seen grazing nearby, while the sky is patrolled by bearded vultures and alpine choughs.

The trail passes through the Segantini Hut, an ideal spot to rest and enjoy the scenery. This hut is named after the famous painter Giovanni Segantini, who found inspiration in these mountains. The trail then continues along a gentle descent back to the funicular station.

Nearby accommodations include the Romantik Hotel Muottas Muragl, located at the top of the funicular, or the Hotel Waldhaus am See at Via Dim Lej 6, 7500 St. Moritz, offering lakeside luxury with convenient access to the trail.

For dining, the Panorama Restaurant at the summit of Muottas Muragl provides exquisite meals with a view, while the Alp Languard Restaurant in Pontresina offers traditional dishes in a charming alpine setting.

Parking is available at the Punt Muragl parking lot, costing CHF 10 per day. GPS coordinates are 46.5215° N, 9.9046° E.

To access the trail, take a train to Pontresina, then a bus, or walk to the Punt Muragl funicular. For guided hikes, consider Engadin Outdoor Center (Address: Via Maistra 41, 7505 Celerina), which offers comprehensive hiking tours in the region.

Schafberg Panorama Trail

The Schafberg Panorama Trail, situated in the Toggenburg region, offers breathtaking views of the Churfirsten mountain range and Lake Walen. This moderate hike covers 8 kilometers (5 miles) and ranges in altitude from 1,378 meters (4,521 feet) to 1,950 meters (6,398 feet), taking about 4 hours to complete.

Starting from the Oberdorf cable car station in Wildhaus, the trail ascends through alpine meadows where you'll encounter wildflowers like alpine asters and monkshood. The path continues to the summit of Schafberg, offering a panoramic vista of the Säntis massif and the rolling hills below. The descent towards the Sellamatt plateau passes through enchanting pine forests, where you might spot roe deer and red squirrels.

Accommodation options include the Hotel Hirschen Wildhaus, located at Dorf 1, 9658 Wildhaus, and the Berggasthaus Oberdorf, situated directly at the cable car station. Both offer comfortable lodgings with easy trail access.

For dining, the Berggasthaus Meglisalp offers hearty alpine cuisine with stunning views, and the Restaurant Toggenburg at Postplatz 27, 9656 Alt St. Johann, serves delicious local dishes.

Parking is available at the Oberdorf cable car station for CHF 5 per day. GPS coordinates are 47.1972° N, 9.3500° E.

To get to the trailhead, take a train to Buchs SG, then a bus to Wildhaus. For a guided hike, Toggenburg Bergführer (Address: Schönenbodensee, 9657 Alt St. Johann) offers professional guiding services.

Five Lakes Hike in Zermatt

The Five Lakes Hike, or 5-Seenweg, in Zermatt, is a picturesque trail that takes you through stunning alpine scenery and past five beautiful lakes. This 9.3-kilometer (5.8 miles) trail, with an altitude range of 2,538 meters (8,327 feet) at its highest point, is moderately challenging and typically takes around 3-4 hours to complete.

The trail starts at Blauherd, reached via a funicular and cable car from Zermatt. The first lake, Stellisee, offers mirror-like reflections of the iconic Matterhorn. The path continues to Grindjisee, where you can observe rare alpine flowers like gentian and mountain avens. Next is Grünsee, surrounded by lush meadows frequented by grazing sheep. Moosjisee, the fourth lake, showcases a stunning turquoise hue due to glacier meltwater. The final lake, Leisee, is a popular spot for a refreshing dip.

Accommodation recommendations include the Hotel Matthiol at Moosstrasse 40, 3920 Zermatt, and the Riffelalp Resort, located at Riffelalp, 3920 Zermatt. Both provide luxury stays with easy access to the hike.

For dining, Restaurant Fluhalp offers traditional Swiss dishes with stunning views of the Matterhorn, and the Findlerhof at Findeln 2051, 3920 Zermatt, serves delicious local cuisine.

Parking in Zermatt is limited to the Täsch parking facility, costing CHF 14 per day. GPS coordinates are 46.0620° N, 7.7797° E. From Täsch, take a shuttle train to Zermatt.

To reach the trailhead, take the funicular from Zermatt to Sunnegga, then transfer to the Blauherd cable car. For guided hikes, Zermatters (Address: Bahnhofplatz 5, 3920 Zermatt) offers experienced guides to enhance your hiking experience.

Mürren to Gimmelwald Via Ferrata

The Mürren to Gimmelwald Via Ferrata offers an exhilarating experience for adventure seekers, combining breathtaking alpine scenery with a thrilling challenge. This unique trail, situated in the Bernese Oberland, features iron rungs, cables, and ladders that guide hikers along steep rock faces. At an altitude of 1,650 meters (5,413 feet) in Mürren, descending to 1,367 meters (4,485 feet) in Gimmelwald, the via ferrata stretches about 2.2 kilometers (1.4 miles) and typically takes 2-3 hours to complete. The difficulty level is high, requiring a good head for heights and proper equipment, including a helmet, harness, and via Ferrata set.

Starting in the picturesque village of Mürren, accessible by train and cable car from Lauterbrunnen, the route quickly engages you with stunning views of the Eiger, Mönch, and Jungfrau peaks. The trail passes through rugged terrain where you'll find alpine flora such as alpine anemones and mountain sorrel. Golden eagles and alpine choughs are common sights, soaring in the skies above. Historical features include the traditional wooden chalets of Mürren and Gimmelwald, embodying the charm of Swiss mountain life.

As the route progresses, you'll encounter a series of thrilling sections, including the famous Nepal Bridge and vertical ladders that require careful navigation. The trail descends gradually into Gimmelwald, a quaint farming village.

Accommodation options include the Hotel Alpenruh at Schilthornbahn AG, 3825 Mürren, and the Pension Gimmelwald, located at Gimmelwald 1487, 3826 Gimmelwald. Both offer cozy lodgings with stunning views.

For dining, consider the Stägerstübli in Gimmelwald, which offers hearty Swiss dishes, or the Eiger Guesthouse in Mürren, located at Aegerten 1079B, 3825 Mürren, known for its delicious local cuisine.

Parking is available at the Lauterbrunnen parking lot, costing around CHF 14 per day. GPS coordinates for the lot are 46.5944° N, 7.9086° E. From Lauterbrunnen, take the cable car to Grütschalp and then the train to Mürren.

To reach the trailhead, travel by train to Lauterbrunnen, then take the cable car and train to Mürren. For a guided experience, consider Klettersteig Mürren-Gimmelwald (Address: Mürren, 3825 Lauterbrunnen) which offers professional guides.

Eiger Trail

The Eiger Trail is a remarkable hike offering stunning views of the north face of the Eiger, one of the most iconic peaks in the Swiss Alps. This trail, stretching from Eigergletscher to Alpiglen, is about 6 kilometers (3.7 miles) long and sits between altitudes of 2,320 meters

(7,612 feet) and 1,615 meters (5,299 feet). Rated as moderate in difficulty, the hike takes approximately 2-3 hours to complete.

The journey begins at the Eigergletscher station, reached via the Jungfraujoch railway. The trail meanders through alpine meadows and rocky paths, offering spectacular views of the Eiger's daunting north face. Along the way, you can spot alpine flora such as edelweiss and alpine asters. Wildlife sightings might include ibex, marmots, and choughs.

Historical points of interest include the infamous Eigerwand station, once used by mountaineers attempting to scale the north face. As the trail descends towards Alpiglen, the vistas of Grindelwald and the surrounding peaks are truly captivating.

Accommodation near the trail includes the Berghaus Alpiglen, located at Alpiglen, 3818 Grindelwald, and the Hotel Glacier, situated at Endweg 55, 3818 Grindelwald. Both offer comfortable lodging with easy access to the trail.

For a bite to eat, Restaurant Alpiglen provides delicious meals right on the trail, while Barry's Restaurant in Grindelwald, located at Dorfstrasse 175, 3818 Grindelwald, offers hearty Swiss cuisine.

Parking is available at the Grindelwald Grund parking lot, costing CHF 5 per day. GPS coordinates are 46.6231° N, 8.0373° E. From Grindelwald, take the Jungfrau railway to Eigergletscher.

To reach the trailhead, take a train to Grindelwald, then board the Jungfraujoch railway to Eigergletscher. For guided hikes, Alpine

Guides Grindelwald (Address: Dorfstrasse 187, 3818 Grindelwald) offers expert-led tours along the Eiger Trail.

Matterhorn Trek

The Matterhorn Trek is an epic adventure for seasoned hikers, offering close encounters with the iconic Matterhorn and the spectacular scenery of the Swiss Alps. This multi-day trek spans approximately 53 kilometers (33 miles), with altitudes ranging from 1,620 meters (5,315 feet) in Zermatt to 3,130 meters (10,270 feet) at the highest point. The trek is rated difficult due to its length and elevation changes, typically taking 4-6 days to complete.

Starting in Zermatt, a picturesque town at the foot of the Matterhorn, the trail winds through lush meadows, pine forests, and rocky landscapes. Notable plants include the vibrant alpine poppy and the rare glacier buttercup. Wildlife sightings might include marmots, chamois, and the elusive alpine ibex. The trail also passes several historical features, such as traditional alpine huts and the historic Hörnli Hut, used by climbers attempting to summit the Matterhorn.

Highlights of the trek include crossing the Theodul Glacier and the stunning views from the Trockener Steg and Schwarzsee stations. Each day brings new vistas and challenges, culminating in breathtaking panoramas of the Matterhorn and surrounding peaks.

Accommodation options along the trek include the Hörnli Hut at Matterhorn, 3920 Zermatt, and the Hotel Schwarzsee, located at Schwarzsee, 3920 Zermatt. Both offer essential amenities for trekkers.

Dining options are limited on the trail, but the Restaurant Furri in Zermatt, located at Furri, 3920 Zermatt, provides hearty meals, and Chez Vrony at Findeln, 3920 Zermatt, offers gourmet alpine cuisine with stunning views.

Parking in Zermatt is limited to the Täsch parking facility, costing CHF 14 per day. GPS coordinates are 46.0620° N, 7.7797° E. From Täsch, take a shuttle train to Zermatt.

To begin the trek, travel to Zermatt by train. For guided treks, Zermatters (Address: Bahnhofplatz 5, 3920 Zermatt) offers professional guides to ensure a safe and enjoyable experience.

Bernese Oberland Traverse

The Bernese Oberland Traverse is a spectacular long-distance hike through some of Switzerland's most stunning landscapes, covering approximately 70 kilometers (43 miles) from Meiringen to Gstaad. The trail ranges in altitude from 595 meters (1,952 feet) in Meiringen to 2,764 meters (9,068 feet) at its highest points, offering a moderate to difficult challenge over 5-7 days.

The route begins in Meiringen, accessible by train, and ascends through lush valleys and rugged mountain passes. Along the way, hikers will encounter a diverse array of flora, including alpine roses and gentians, as well as fauna such as chamois and golden eagles. The trail also passes historical sites like the Rosenlaui Glacier Gorge and the picturesque village of Grindelwald.

Key highlights include crossing the Grosse Scheidegg pass, with its stunning views of the Eiger, and the descent into Lauterbrunnen Valley, famed for its 72 waterfalls. The trail continues through Wengen, over the Kleine Scheidegg, and down into Grindelwald. Each segment offers unique landscapes and challenges, culminating in the beautiful town of Gstaad.

Accommodations include the Hotel Victoria Jungfrau, located at Höheweg 41, 3800 Interlaken, and the Gstaad Palace at Palacestrasse 28, 3780 Gstaad. Both offer luxurious stays with access to the trail.

Dining options are plentiful in the towns along the route, with Restaurant Golden India in Interlaken (Höheweg 135, 3800 Interlaken) offering delicious meals, and Restaurant Gstaaderhof (Lauenenstrasse 19, 3780 Gstaad) providing traditional Swiss cuisine.

Parking is available at the Meiringen parking facility for CHF 10 per day. GPS coordinates are 46.7265° N, and 8.1831° E. From Meiringen, take the train to the trailhead.

To access the trail, take a train to Meiringen. For guided hikes, Alpinehikers (Address: Meiringen, 3860 Meiringen) offers expert-led tours along the Bernese Oberland Traverse.

Via Alpina

The Via Alpina is a remarkable long-distance hiking trail that traverses the heart of the Swiss Alps, offering a deep dive into Switzerland's stunning natural landscapes, diverse flora and fauna, and rich cultural history. Stretching over 390 kilometers (242 miles) and encompassing an altitude range from 500 meters (1,640 feet) to 2,800 meters (9,186 feet), the trail is divided into 20 stages, each varying in difficulty from moderate to challenging. Hikers typically complete the entire route in about three weeks, although it can be divided into shorter sections.

Starting in Vaduz, Liechtenstein, and ending in Montreux, Switzerland, the trail passes through several iconic Swiss regions, including the Bernese Oberland and the Valais. The route takes you through lush meadows, dense forests, and rugged mountain passes, with highlights such as the Engstligen Falls and the scenic village of Kandersteg. Along the way, hikers can spot alpine flora like edelweiss and gentians, and wildlife such as marmots, ibex, and golden eagles.

Key stages include the ascent to the Hohtürli Pass, offering panoramic views of the Blüemlisalp glacier, and the traverse of the historic Gemmi Pass, with its dramatic cliffs and sweeping vistas. Each stage offers unique landscapes and cultural experiences, from traditional Swiss chalets to ancient alpine traditions.

Accommodations along the Via Alpina include the charming Hotel Adler in Kandersteg, located at Äussere Dorfstrasse 19, 3718 Kandersteg, and the cozy Hotel Bellevue des Alpes at Kleine Scheidegg, 3823 Lauterbrunnen. Both provide comfortable lodging and easy access to the trail.

For dining, the Restaurant Doldenhorn in Kandersteg (Äussere Dorfstrasse 40, 3718 Kandersteg) offers gourmet Swiss cuisine, while the Berghaus Bäregg in Grindelwald (Postfach 110, 3818 Grindelwald) serves hearty alpine dishes with stunning views.

Parking is available at the trail's various starting points, with costs varying by location. For example, parking in Kandersteg costs around CHF 5 per day. GPS coordinates for Kandersteg parking are 46.4953° N, 7.6731° E.

To start the trail, take a train to Vaduz, Liechtenstein. For guided hikes, consider Alpinehikers (Address: Grindelwaldstrasse 19, 3818 Grindelwald), offering expert-led tours along the Via Alpina.

Brienzer Rothorn Panorama Trail

The Brienzer Rothorn Panorama Trail is a scenic hike in the Bernese Oberland, offering panoramic views of Lake Brienz and the surrounding Alps. This 12-kilometer (7.5 miles) trail starts at the Brienzer Rothorn, which can be reached by a historic steam cogwheel train from Brienz, and descends to Planalp. The trail ranges from an altitude of 2,350 meters (7,710 feet) at the Rothorn to 1,340 meters (4,396 feet) at Planalp, presenting a moderate challenge that takes about 4-5 hours to complete.

Starting at the summit of the Brienzer Rothorn, hikers are treated to sweeping views of Lake Brienz and the Bernese Alps, including peaks like the Eiger, Mönch, and Jungfrau. The trail winds through alpine meadows dotted with wildflowers such as alpine asters and gentians. Along the way, you might spot chamois, marmots, and soaring birds of prey like golden eagles.

As you descend, the trail passes through lush forests and open meadows, with several viewpoints offering breathtaking vistas of the turquoise waters of Lake Brienz. Historical features include the charming alpine huts and traditional Swiss chalets scattered along the route.

Accommodation options near the trail include the Grandhotel Giessbach, located at Axalpstrasse, 3855 Brienz, and the Hotel Brienzerburli, situated at Hauptstrasse 11, 3855 Brienz. Both provide comfortable lodging with easy access to the trail.

For dining, the Berghaus Planalp offers delicious local cuisine with a scenic terrace, and the Restaurant Steinbock in Brienz, located at Hauptstrasse 123, 3855 Brienz, serves traditional Swiss dishes.

Parking is available at the Brienz Rothorn Bahn station, costing around CHF 5 per day. GPS coordinates for the parking lot are 46.7540° N, 8.0507° E.

To reach the trailhead, take the cogwheel train from Brienz to the summit of the Brienzer Rothorn. For a guided hike, consider Outdoor Interlaken (Address: Hauptstrasse 15, 3800 Interlaken), which offers guided tours of the Brienzer Rothorn area.

Pizol 5-Lakes Hike

The Pizol 5-Lakes Hike is a stunning high-altitude trail in eastern Switzerland, renowned for its five crystal-clear alpine lakes. This 10.6-kilometer (6.6 miles) loop trail starts and ends at the Pizolhütte, with an altitude range from 2,222 meters (7,290 feet) to 2,844 meters (9,331 feet), offering a moderate challenge that typically takes about 4-5 hours to complete.

Beginning at the Pizolhütte, reached by a cable car from Wangs, the trail quickly ascends to the first lake, Wildsee, surrounded by rugged peaks and meadows. Continuing, you'll encounter the tranquil Schottensee, reflecting the surrounding mountains. Next is the milky-blue Schwarzsee, followed by the deep green Baschalvasee. The final lake, Wangsersee, marks the descent back to the Pizolhütte.

The trail offers breathtaking alpine scenery, with diverse flora such as edelweiss and alpine roses. Wildlife enthusiasts may spot marmots, chamois, and even the occasional ibex. Historical features include remnants of old shepherd huts and alpine farming structures.

Accommodation options include the Pizolhütte itself, located at Bergstation Laufböden, 7323 Wangs, and the Hotel Schloss Ragaz at Schloss-Strasse, 7310 Bad Ragaz, offering comfortable stays with easy access to the trail.

For dining, the Bergrestaurant Pizolhütte provides hearty meals with panoramic views, and the Restaurant Alpenrose in Wangs, located at Dorfstrasse 19, 7323 Wangs, offers traditional Swiss dishes.

Parking is available at the Pizolbahn cable car station in Wangs, costing around CHF 5 per day. GPS coordinates are 46.9860° N, 9.4347° E.

To reach the trailhead, take the cable car from Wangs to the Pizolhütte. For a guided experience, consider Swiss Trekking Tours (Address: Bahnhofstrasse 8, 7320 Sargans), offering expert-led hikes in the Pizol region.

Gornergrat Panorama Trail

The Gornergrat Panorama Trail offers hikers spectacular views of the Matterhorn and the surrounding Alpine peaks. This 6.7-kilometer (4.2 miles) trail starts at the Gornergrat railway station, descending to Riffelberg. The trail ranges in altitude from 3,089 meters (10,135 feet) at Gornergrat to 2,582 meters (8,471 feet) at Riffelberg, providing a moderate hike that takes about 2-3 hours.

Beginning at the Gornergrat railway station, accessible by the Gornergrat Bahn from Zermatt, the trail immediately offers panoramic views of the Matterhorn, Monte Rosa, and the Gorner Glacier. The path winds through alpine meadows and rocky terrain, adorned with wildflowers like alpine poppies and gentians. Wildlife sightings might include ibex, marmots, and the occasional golden eagle.

As you descend, the trail offers breathtaking vistas of the surrounding peaks and the Gorner Glacier. Historical features along the route include the historic Riffelberg Hotel and remnants of old alpine farming structures.

Accommodation options near the trail include the 3100 Kulmhotel Gornergrat, located at Gornergrat, 3920 Zermatt, and the Riffelhaus 1853, situated at Riffelberg, 3920 Zermatt. Both offer comfortable lodging with stunning views.

For dining, the Restaurant 3100 Kulmhotel provides gourmet meals with panoramic views, and the Restaurant Alphitta on Riffelberg, located at Riffelberg, 3920 Zermatt, offers traditional Swiss cuisine.

Parking is available at the Täsch parking facility, costing CHF 14 per day. GPS coordinates are 46.0620° N, 7.7797° E. From Täsch, take a shuttle train to Zermatt.

To reach the trailhead, take the Gornergrat Bahn from Zermatt to the Gornergrat railway station. For guided hikes, consider Zermatters (Address: Bahnhofplatz 5, 3920 Zermatt), offering professional guides to enhance your hiking experience.

Aletsch Glacier Panorama Trail

The Aletsch Glacier Panorama Trail offers an unforgettable hiking experience, presenting a sweeping view of the largest glacier in the Alps. This trail begins at Bettmerhorn and winds its way to Riederalp, spanning approximately 12 kilometers (7.5 miles) with an altitude range from 2,647 meters (8,684 feet) at Bettmerhorn to 1,925 meters (6,316 feet) at Riederalp. Rated as moderate in difficulty, it typically takes around 4-5 hours to complete.

The trail starts at the Bettmerhorn, accessible via cable car from Bettmeralp. From here, you're greeted with a majestic view of the Aletsch Glacier, a UNESCO World Heritage site. The trail follows the glacier's edge, providing breathtaking panoramas of the vast ice field and surrounding peaks like the Eiger, Mönch, and Jungfrau. Alpine flora such as edelweiss, alpine roses, and gentians dot the path, and wildlife sightings might include chamois, marmots, and the rare bearded vulture.

Historical features include the Aletsch Forest, one of the oldest in Switzerland, and the Villa Cassel, a historic mansion now serving as a nature conservation center. The trail meanders through lush meadows, rocky outcrops, and ancient forests, offering a diverse and captivating landscape.

For accommodation, consider the Hotel Waldhaus in Bettmeralp, located at Bettmeralp, 3992 Bettmeralp, and the Berghotel Riederfurka at Riederalp, 3987 Riederalp. Both provide cozy lodging with easy access to the trail.

Dining options include Restaurant Bettmerhof in Bettmeralp (Address: Bettmeralp 3992) for a taste of traditional Swiss cuisine, and Restaurant Alpenglück in Riederalp (Address: Riederalp 3987) offering hearty alpine dishes.

Parking is available at the Betten Talstation for about CHF 8 per day. GPS coordinates are 46.3574° N, 8.0566° E. From there, take the cable car to Bettmeralp and then a second cable car to Bettmerhorn.

To reach the trailhead, travel by train to Betten Talstation, then take the cable car to Bettmeralp and subsequently to Bettmerhorn. For guided hikes, consider hiring a local guide from Aletsch Arena (Address: Furkastrasse 39, 3983 Mörel).

Schönbühl Panorama Trail

The Schönbühl Panorama Trail offers a picturesque hike through the Swiss Prealps, featuring stunning views of Lake Thun and the surrounding mountains. This trail, starting from Beatenberg and ending at Habkern, covers about 8 kilometers (5 miles) with altitudes ranging from 1,650 meters (5,413 feet) at Beatenberg to 1,100 meters (3,609 feet) at Habkern. The trail is moderately challenging and takes around 3-4 hours to complete.

Starting in Beatenberg, accessible by bus from Interlaken, the trail ascends gently through alpine meadows and forests. The route offers sweeping views of Lake Thun and the Bernese Alps, with notable peaks like the Eiger, Mönch, and Jungfrau visible on clear days. Along the way, hikers can admire alpine flora such as gentians, orchids, and buttercups, while keeping an eye out for local wildlife like ibex, roe deer, and golden eagles.

One of the trail's highlights is the panoramic viewpoint at Schönbühl, offering an unobstructed view of Lake Thun and the surrounding mountains. Historical features along the route include traditional Swiss chalets and alpine farms that provide a glimpse into the region's pastoral heritage.

Accommodation options include Hotel Beausite Beatenberg, located at Mauren 555, 3803 Beatenberg, and Hotel Bären in Habkern at Postgasse, 3804 Habkern. Both offer comfortable stays with easy access to the trail.

For dining, Restaurant Alpenblick in Beatenberg (Address: Mauren 556, 3803 Beatenberg) offers delicious Swiss dishes, while Restaurant Chemihütte in Habkern (Address: Schwanden 258A, 3804 Habkern) serves traditional meals in a rustic setting.

Parking is available at the Beatenberg station for about CHF 5 per day. GPS coordinates are 46.6860° N, 7.7946° E.

To reach the trailhead, take a train to Interlaken, then a bus to Beatenberg. For guided hikes, contact Swiss Alpine Guides (Address: Hauptstrasse 15, 3800 Interlaken) for professional guidance.

First to Bachalpsee Trail

The First to Bachalpsee Trail is a beloved hiking route in the Bernese Oberland, known for its idyllic alpine lake and spectacular mountain vistas. The trail starts at First, reachable by a gondola from Grindelwald, and leads to Bachalpsee, then back to First, covering approximately 6 kilometers (3.7 miles) round-trip. With an altitude of 2,167 meters (7,109 feet) at First and 2,265 meters (7,431 feet) at Bachalpsee, it is an easy to moderate hike that takes about 2-3 hours.

Beginning at First, the trail meanders through alpine meadows adorned with wildflowers such as alpine roses and gentians. The path is well-maintained and offers breathtaking views of the surrounding peaks, including the Wetterhorn, Schreckhorn, and Finsteraarhorn. Wildlife enthusiasts might spot marmots, alpine choughs, and occasionally ibex.

The highlight of the trail is Bachalpsee, a pristine alpine lake reflecting the snow-capped peaks in its crystal-clear waters. It's a perfect spot for a rest and picnic, offering stunning photo opportunities. The trail is family-friendly and well-suited for hikers of all ages.

Accommodation options include the Hotel Belvedere Grindelwald, located at Dorfstrasse 53, 3818 Grindelwald, and the Hotel Gletschergarten at Obere Gletscherstrasse 1, 3818 Grindelwald. Both provide comfortable lodgings with scenic views and convenient access to the gondola.

For dining, consider Restaurant First Mountain, right at the gondola station, for a meal with a view, and Restaurant Alpenblick in Grindelwald (Address: Obere Gletscherstrasse 16, 3818 Grindelwald) for traditional Swiss fare.

Parking is available at the Grindelwald Firstbahn parking lot, costing around CHF 5 per day. GPS coordinates are 46.6244° N, 8.0422° E.

To reach the trailhead, take a train to Grindelwald, then the gondola to First. For guided hikes, contact Grindelwald Tourism (Address: Dorfstrasse 110, 3818 Grindelwald) for expert-led tours.

Schilthorn Panorama Trail

The Schilthorn Panorama Trail offers a breathtaking hike with views of the Eiger, Mönch, and Jungfrau. Starting at the Schilthorn summit, reached via cable car from Mürren, the trail descends to Birg and then to Mürren, covering about 8 kilometers (5 miles) with an altitude range from 2,970 meters (9,744 feet) at Schilthorn to 1,638 meters (5,374 feet) at Mürren. The hike is moderately challenging and takes around 4-5 hours to complete.

From the Schilthorn, famous for its revolving restaurant and James Bond connections, the trail offers stunning panoramic views. The descent to Birg takes you through rocky paths and alpine meadows filled with wildflowers such as edelweiss and alpine asters. Keep an eye out for wildlife like ibex, marmots, and golden eagles soaring above.

The trail continues from Birg to Mürren, passing through lush meadows and offering views of the Lauterbrunnen Valley. Historical points of interest include the old Schilthorn cable car station and Mürren's traditional wooden chalets.

Accommodation options in Mürren include the Hotel Alpenruh, located at Schilthornbahn AG, 3825 Mürren, and the Hotel Eiger, situated at Aegerten 1079B, 3825 Mürren. Both offer cozy stays with spectacular views.

For dining, the Piz Gloria Restaurant at the Schilthorn Summit provides a unique dining experience with 360-degree views, and the Eiger Guesthouse in Mürren offers delicious local cuisine.

Parking is available at the Stechelberg cable car station, costing about CHF 8 per day. GPS coordinates are 46.5633° N, 7.8991° E. From Stechelberg, take the cable car to Mürren, then transfer to the Schilthornbahn.

To reach the trailhead, take a train to Lauterbrunnen, then a bus to Stechelberg, followed by a cable car ride to Schilthorn. For guided hikes, consider Mountain Guide Mürren (Address: 3825 Mürren), offering professional guidance and safety.

Saas-Fee to Saas-Grund Trail

The Saas-Fee to Saas-Grund Trail is a delightful hike through the heart of the Swiss Alps, offering picturesque views and an intimate look at alpine life. Spanning approximately 6 kilometers (3.7 miles), with an altitude range from 1,800 meters (5,906 feet) in Saas-Fee to 1,550 meters (5,085 feet) in Saas-Grund, this trail is moderately difficult and typically takes around 2-3 hours to complete.

The hike begins in Saas-Fee, a charming car-free village surrounded by towering peaks and lush green valleys. As you set off, the path takes you through verdant alpine meadows, where you might spot gentians and alpine roses in bloom. Keep an eye out for chamois and marmots as you walk along the well-marked trail.

As you descend towards Saas-Grund, the route meanders through traditional Swiss villages and dense forests. These forests are home to a variety of wildlife, and if you're lucky, you might catch sight of a golden eagle soaring above. The trail also offers stunning views of the Dom, the highest mountain entirely in Switzerland.

For accommodations, consider the cozy Hotel Alpenperle in Saas-Fee (Dorfstrasse 99, 3906 Saas-Fee) or the welcoming Hotel Alpha in Saas-Grund (Unter dem Berg 1, 3910 Saas-Grund). Both offer comfortable rooms and easy access to the trail.

When it's time to eat, Restaurant Tenne in Saas-Fee (Obere Dorfstrasse 64, 3906 Saas-Fee) and Restaurant Del Ponte in Saas-Grund (Dorfplatz, 3910 Saas-Grund) serve up hearty mountain cuisine that will satisfy any hiker's appetite.

Parking is available in Saas-Fee at several locations, with costs depending on the duration of your stay. For example, Parking Haus Saas Fee (46.1092° N, 7.9272° E) offers convenient access.

To reach the trailhead, take a train to Visp and then transfer to a bus bound for Saas-Fee. The trailhead starts in the village center, making it easy to find your way.

For those seeking a guided hiking experience, Alpine Adventures Saas-Fee (Obere Dorfstrasse 64, 3906 Saas-Fee) offers expert-led tours through the region's stunning landscapes.

Aletsch Forest Trail

The Aletsch Forest Trail takes you through one of Europe's most pristine and ancient forests. This 10-kilometer (6.2 miles) hike, with altitudes ranging from 1,800 meters (5,906 feet) to 2,300 meters (7,546 feet), is moderately challenging and offers an extraordinary natural experience.

The trail starts in Fiescheralp, accessible by a scenic cable car ride from Fiesch. As you hike through the dense forest of towering Swiss pines and spruces, the tranquility is broken only by the sounds of birds and the occasional rustle of wildlife. Keep an eye out for rare orchids and the elusive red deer that roam these woods.

The route offers breathtaking views of the Aletsch Glacier, the largest glacier in the Alps. Along the trail, you'll find interpretive signs explaining the unique geological features and the history of this ancient landscape. The Aletsch Forest itself is a UNESCO World Heritage site, protecting a rich biodiversity.

For a comfortable stay, Hotel Alpina in Fiesch (Gletscherstube 2, 3984 Fiesch) and Hotel La Collina in Fiescheralp (Fiescheralp, 3984 Fiescheralp) offer excellent accommodations.

After your hike, enjoy a meal at Restaurant Pizzeria Al Ponte in Fiesch (Kirchweg 1, 3984 Fiesch) or Restaurant Bergfreund in Fiescheralp (Fiescheralp, 3984 Fiescheralp).

Parking in Fiesch is available at various locations, such as Parking Zentrum (46.4044° N, 8.1356° E), with costs depending on the duration.

To get to the trailhead, take a train to Fiesch, then the Fiesch-Eggishorn cable car to Fiescheralp. The trail begins at the top of the lift.

For guided tours, contact Swiss Mountain Guide (Kirchweg 9, 3984 Fiesch), known for their knowledgeable guides and engaging tours.

Zermatt Five-Seenweg (Five Lakes Trail)

The Five-Seenweg, or Five Lakes Trail, near Zermatt, is a picturesque hike that passes five stunning alpine lakes. This 9-kilometer (5.6 miles) trail, with altitudes ranging from 2,200 meters (7,218 feet) to 2,500 meters (8,202 feet), is moderately challenging and takes about 3-4 hours to complete.

The hike starts from Sunnegga, reached by funicular from Zermatt. The first lake, Leisee, offers clear waters perfect for a refreshing dip. Moving on to Grindjisee, you'll find it surrounded by vibrant meadows and offering views of the Matterhorn. Stellisee is next, famous for its perfect reflections of the iconic peak, making it a favorite spot for photographers.

As you continue, Grünsee offers a serene setting with scattered larch trees, and finally, Moosjisee's turquoise waters, colored by glacier minerals, provide a stunning end to the journey. Along the way, watch for ibex, marmots, and the diverse alpine flora, including edelweiss.

For accommodations, Hotel Bellerive (Riedstrasse 3, 3920 Zermatt) and Hotel Alex (Bodmenstrasse 12, 3920 Zermatt) are excellent choices.

After the hike, savor a meal at Restaurant Chez Vrony (Findeln, 3920 Zermatt) or Restaurant Stellisee (Stelliseeweg, 3920 Zermatt).

Parking in Zermatt is limited since it's a car-free village, but you can park in Täsch and take a shuttle to Zermatt. Parking at Matterhorn Terminal Täsch (46.0645° N, 7.7766° E) is a convenient option.

To reach the trailhead, take a train to Zermatt and then the Sunnegga funicular.

For guided hikes, contact Zermatt Active (Bahnhofplatz 5, 3920 Zermatt), offering a range of tours, including the Five Lakes Trail.

Gemmi Pass Trail

The Gemmi Pass Trail is a historic route connecting the cantons of Valais and Bern, offering spectacular views of the Swiss Alps. The 8-kilometer (5 miles) trail, with altitudes ranging from 1,500 meters (4,921 feet) to 2,340 meters (7,677 feet), is moderately to highly challenging and takes about 3-4 hours to complete.

Starting in Leukerbad, the trail climbs steadily towards the Gemmi Pass. Along the way, you'll pass alpine meadows bursting with wildflowers and traditional wooden chalets. As you reach higher altitudes, the views of the Rhône Valley and the Bernese Alps are breathtaking.

Crossing the historic Gemmi Pass, once a vital trade route, is a highlight. The trail then descends towards Kandersteg, passing the serene Daubensee lake. The forested descent offers shade and the chance to spot local wildlife like marmots and golden eagles.

For accommodations, consider Hotel de France (Rathausstrasse 51, 3954 Leukerbad) or Gemmi Lodge (Gemmiweg, 3718 Kandersteg).

After the hike, enjoy a meal at Restaurant Panorama (Gemmiweg, 3718 Kandersteg) or Bergrestaurant Schwarenbach (Schwarenbach, 3718 Kandersteg).

Parking is available in Leukerbad and Kandersteg. For example, Parking Leukerbad Therme (46.3772° N, 7.6296° E) is a good option.

To reach the trailhead, take a train to Leukerbad. The trail begins in the village center.

For guided tours, contact Outdoor Interlaken (Hauptstrasse 15, 3800 Interlaken), known for their comprehensive guided hiking experiences.

Chapter 4

Difficult Trails (For Experienced Hikers and Mountaineers)

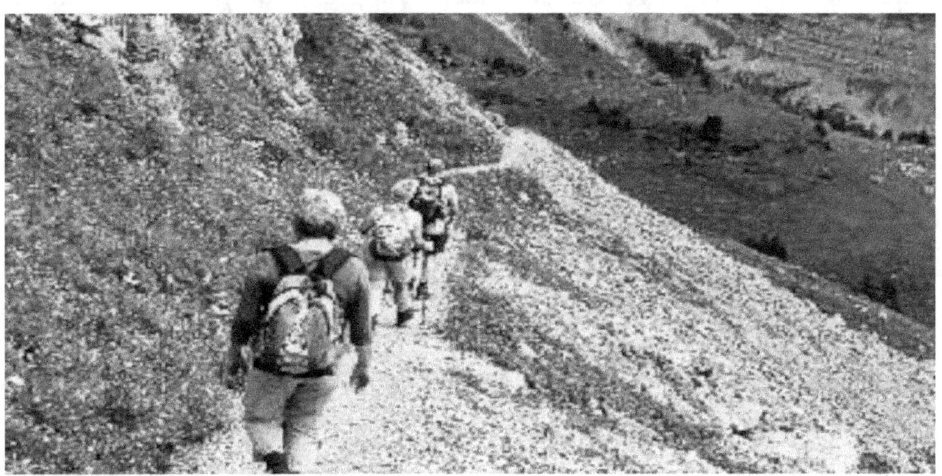

The Haute Route

The Haute Route, also known as the High Route or Mountaineers' Route, is a classic trek that traverses the stunning landscapes of the Swiss Alps, connecting the two mountain resorts of Chamonix in France and Zermatt in Switzerland. This iconic trail offers hikers the opportunity to experience some of the most spectacular scenery in the Alps, including towering peaks, vast glaciers, and picturesque alpine villages. As you hike the Haute Route, you'll encounter a diverse range of flora and fauna, from colorful wildflowers and fragrant pine forests to elusive mountain ibex and chamois. Along the way, you'll also discover historic mountain huts, remote alpine lakes, and ancient footpaths that have been used by generations of mountain travelers.

Altitude, Length, and Difficulty Level

The Haute Route covers a distance of approximately 180 kilometers (112 miles) and typically takes between 10 to 14 days to complete, depending on the specific route and itinerary chosen. The trail traverses high mountain passes, steep rocky terrain, and snow-covered glaciers, making it suitable for experienced hikers with a good level of fitness and mountain trekking experience.

Route, Distance, Time, and Grade

The Haute Route follows a well-marked route that ascends and descends through the heart of the Alps, crossing several high mountain passes and cols along the way. A typical day on the trail may cover a distance of 10 to 20 kilometers (6 to 12 miles) and take between 6 to 8 hours to complete, including breaks and rest stops. The terrain varies from moderate to strenuous, with sections of rocky terrain, exposed ridges, and steep ascents.

Hiking Regulations

Due to the challenging nature of the Haute Route, it is not recommended for beginners or inexperienced hikers. Pets are generally not allowed on this trail due to the hazardous terrain and potential dangers posed by high altitudes and extreme weather conditions. Hikers are advised to check local weather forecasts and trail conditions before embarking on the hike and to be prepared for changing conditions at high elevations.

Closest Accommodation: (Cabane de Dix: Val d'Hérens, 1984 La Forclaz. Situated at an altitude of 2,928 meters (9,606 feet), this mountain hut offers basic accommodation and stunning views of the surrounding peaks.), **(Hotel Weisshorn**: 3961 St. Luc. Nestled in the heart of the Valais Alps, this historic hotel provides comfortable rooms and traditional Swiss hospitality, making it an ideal base for exploring the region.)

Closest Places to Eat: (Restaurant La Cabane: Route de Mollens 100, 3961 St. Luc. This cozy restaurant serves hearty Swiss cuisine and homemade specialties, perfect for refueling after a day on the trail.) (**Auberge de la Forclaz**: La Forclaz, 1984 La Forclaz. Located near the Cabane de Dix, this rustic inn offers delicious alpine dishes and refreshing beverages, with outdoor seating overlooking the mountains.)

Logistics Upon Arrival

Parking is available in Chamonix and Zermatt at designated parking areas, with daily rates typically ranging from €10 to €20. Alternatively, visitors can reach both towns by train or bus from major cities like Geneva and Zurich, with regular services running throughout the day.

Directions

By Car: From Geneva or Zurich, take the A1 motorway to Martigny, then follow signs for Chamonix or Zermatt, depending on your chosen starting point for the hike. Park in one of the designated parking areas in the town and proceed to the trailhead by foot or public transport.

By Train: Direct trains run from Geneva or Zurich to Martigny, where you can transfer to regional trains or buses bound for Chamonix or Zermatt. From there, follow signs to the Haute Route trailhead.

The Alpine Pass Route

The Alpine Pass Route is a classic trek that crosses the Swiss Alps from east to west, connecting the towns of Sargans in the east to Montreux on the shores of Lake Geneva in the west. This legendary trail offers hikers the opportunity to experience the diverse landscapes and cultural heritage of Switzerland, from rugged mountain passes to lush alpine meadows. While hiking, you'll encounter a variety of plant life, including alpine wildflowers, herbs, and grasses, as well as wildlife such as marmots, mountain goats, and golden eagles. The trail also passes through historic villages, ancient ruins, and traditional alpine farms, providing insight into the region's rich history and cultural traditions.

Altitude, Length, and Difficulty Level

The Alpine Pass Route covers a distance of approximately 350 kilometers (217 miles) and typically takes between 15 to 20 days to complete, depending on the specific route and pace of the hiker. The trail ascends and descends over numerous mountain passes and cols, with elevations ranging from 600 meters (1,968 feet) to over 2,500 meters (8,200 feet) above sea level. The difficulty level varies from moderate to strenuous, with long days of hiking and challenging terrain.

Route, Distance, Time, and Grade

The Alpine Pass Route follows a well-marked trail that winds its way through the heart of the Swiss Alps, crossing over 16 mountain passes and cols along the way. A typical day on the trail may cover a distance of 15 to 25 kilometers (9 to 15 miles) and take between 7 to 10 hours to complete, including breaks and rest stops. The terrain varies from gentle forest paths to rocky mountain trails, with sections of steep ascents and descents.

Hiking Regulations

Pets are generally allowed on the Alpine Pass Route but should be kept on a leash and under control at all times, especially in areas with livestock or wildlife. Hikers are also encouraged to follow Leave No Trace principles, respecting the natural environment and minimizing their impact on the trails.

Closest Accommodation: (Hotel Alpenrose: 7326 Flims Dorf. Situated in the picturesque village of Flims, this cozy hotel offers comfortable rooms and stunning views of the surrounding mountains.) **(Berghotel Tschingelhorn**: Tschingelhornstrasse 5, 3715 Adelboden. Located in the heart of Adelboden, this traditional mountain hotel provides rustic accommodation and easy access to the trailhead.)

Closest Places to Eat: (Restaurant Flims Alpenblick: Via Nova 32, 7017 Flims Dorf. This family-run restaurant serves delicious Swiss cuisine and homemade specialties, with outdoor seating overlooking the mountains.) (Gasthaus Baumgarten: Tschingelhornstrasse 3, 3715 Adelboden. Nestled in the charming village of Adelboden, this cozy Gasthaus offers authentic Swiss dishes and hearty mountain fare, perfect for replenishing energy after a day on the trail.)

Logistics Upon Arrival

Parking is available in Flims and Adelboden at designated parking areas, with daily rates typically ranging from CHF 10 to CHF 20. Alternatively, visitors can reach both towns by train or bus from major cities like Zurich and Bern, with regular services running throughout the day.

Directions

By Car: From Zurich or Bern, take the A13 motorway to Chur, then follow signs for Flims or Adelboden, depending on your chosen starting point for the hike. Park in one of the designated parking areas in the town and proceed to the trailhead by foot or public transport. **By Train**: Direct trains run from Zurich or Bern to Chur, where you can transfer to regional trains or buses bound for Flims or Adelboden. From there, follow signs to the Alpine Pass Route trailhead.

Recommended Hiking Guide Company

For those seeking guided hikes along the Alpine Pass Route, consider **Swiss Trails**. They offer experienced guides who are knowledgeable about the route and can provide support services, such as luggage transfers and accommodation bookings, to make your trekking experience seamless.

The Via Alpina

The Via Alpina is a long-distance hiking trail that spans eight countries in the heart of the Alps, including Switzerland. The Swiss section of the trail offers hikers the chance to explore some of the most scenic and diverse landscapes in the country, from pristine alpine meadows to rugged mountain peaks. The trail has a wealth of natural beauty and cultural heritage, including towering mountains, sparkling lakes, and charming alpine villages. Keep an eye out for alpine wildlife such as ibex, chamois, and marmots, as well as rare plant species that thrive in the high-altitude environment.

Altitude, Length, and Difficulty Level

The Swiss section of the Via Alpina covers a distance of approximately 390 kilometers (242 miles) and typically takes between 20 to 30 days to complete, depending on the specific route and itinerary chosen. The trail ascends and descends over numerous mountain passes and cols, with elevations ranging from 600 meters (1,968 feet) to over 3,000 meters (9,840 feet) above sea level. The difficulty level varies from moderate to strenuous, with long days of hiking and challenging terrain.

Route, Distance, Time, and Grade

The Via Alpina follows a well-marked route that winds its way through the heart of the Swiss Alps, passing through a variety of landscapes and ecosystems along the way. A typical day on the trail may cover a distance of 15 to 25 kilometers (9 to 15 miles) and take between 7 to 10 hours to complete, including breaks and rest stops. The terrain varies from gentle forest paths to rocky mountain trails, with sections of steep ascents and descents.

Hiking Regulations

Pets are generally allowed on the Via Alpina but should be kept on a leash and under control at all times, especially in areas with livestock or wildlife. Hikers are also encouraged to follow Leave No Trace principles, respecting the natural environment and minimizing their impact on the trails.

Closest Accommodation: (Hotel Bellevue: Dorfstrasse 26, 3818 Grindelwald. Situated in the heart of Grindelwald, this traditional hotel offers comfortable rooms and stunning views of the Eiger, making it an ideal base for exploring the region.) (**Berghotel Faulhorn**: Faulhornweg, 3818 Grindelwald. Located at an altitude of 2,681 meters (8,796 feet), this historic mountain hotel provides rustic accommodation and direct access to the trail, allowing hikers to start their adventure right from the doorstep.)

Closest Places to Eat: (Restaurant Eigerblick: Dorfstrasse 115, 3818 Grindelwald. This cozy restaurant serves delicious Swiss cuisine and homemade desserts, with panoramic views of the surrounding mountains.) (**Berghaus Bort**: Bortweg 2, 3818 Grindelwald. Nestled in the alpine meadows above Grindelwald, this traditional mountain inn offers hearty mountain fare and refreshing beverages, perfect for refueling after a day on the trail.)

Logistics Upon Arrival

Parking is available in Grindelwald at designated parking areas, with daily rates typically ranging from CHF 10 to CHF 20. Alternatively, visitors can reach Grindelwald by train from major cities like Zurich and Interlaken, with regular services running throughout the day.

Directions

By Car: From Zurich or Interlaken, take the A8 motorway to Interlaken, then follow signs for Grindelwald. Park in one of the designated parking areas in the town and proceed to the trailhead by foot or public transport.

By Train: Direct trains run from Zurich or Interlaken to Grindelwald, with a travel time of approximately 2 to 3 hours. From the train station, follow signs to the Via Alpina trailhead.

The Tour du Mont Blanc

The Tour du Mont Blanc is one of the most iconic long-distance hiking trails in the world, circumnavigating the majestic Mont Blanc massif through France, Italy, and Switzerland. This legendary trek offers hikers the opportunity to experience stunning alpine scenery, charming mountain villages, and diverse ecosystems as they traverse the rugged terrain of the Alps. As you hike the Tour du Mont Blanc, you'll encounter a wealth of natural beauty and cultural heritage, from verdant valleys and cascading waterfalls to towering glaciers and snow-capped peaks. Keep an eye out for alpine flora such as edelweiss and gentian, as well as wildlife including ibex, chamois, and marmots. Along the way, you'll also discover historic chalets, rustic mountain huts, and picturesque hamlets that offer insight into the region's rich history and traditions.

Altitude, Length, and Difficulty Level

The Tour du Mont Blanc covers a distance of approximately 170 kilometers (106 miles) and typically takes between 7 to 10 days to complete, depending on the specific route and itinerary chosen. The trail traverses high mountain passes, rocky terrain, and steep ascents, with elevations ranging from 1,000 meters (3,280 feet) to over 2,500 meters (8,200 feet) above sea level. The difficulty level varies from moderate to strenuous, with long days of hiking and challenging terrain.

Route, Distance, Time, and Grade

The Tour du Mont Blanc follows a well-marked route that encircles the Mont Blanc massif, passing through France, Italy, and Switzerland. A typical day on the trail may cover a distance of 15 to 20 kilometers (9 to 12 miles) and take between 6 to 8 hours to complete, including breaks and rest stops. The terrain varies from gentle forest paths to rocky mountain trails, with sections of steep ascents and descents.

Hiking Regulations

Pets are generally allowed on the Tour du Mont Blanc but should be kept on a leash and under control at all times, especially in areas with livestock or wildlife. Hikers are also encouraged to follow Leave No Trace principles, respecting the natural environment and minimizing their impact on the trails.

Closest Accommodation: (Refuge du Col de Balme: Route du Col de Balme, 74400 Vallorcine, France. Situated on the border between France and Switzerland, this mountain refuge offers basic accommodation and stunning views of the surrounding peaks.) **(Hotel La Chaumière**: Via Passerin d'Entreves 5, 11013 Courmayeur, Italy. Located in the charming town of Courmayeur, this cozy hotel provides comfortable rooms and easy access to the trailhead.)

Closest Places to Eat: (Le Refuge des Mottets: Les Mottets, 73700 Bourg-Saint-Maurice, France. This rustic mountain refuge serves hearty alpine cuisine and homemade specialties, with outdoor seating overlooking the Mont Blanc massif.). **(Ristorante Al Caminetto**: Strada Regionale 47, 11013 Courmayeur, Italy. Nestled in the heart of Courmayeur, this traditional Italian restaurant offers delicious pasta dishes, wood-fired pizzas, and local wines.)

Logistics Upon Arrival

Parking is available in Vallorcine and Courmayeur at designated parking areas, with daily rates typically ranging from €10 to €20. Alternatively, visitors can reach both towns by train or bus from major cities like Geneva and Turin, with regular services running throughout the day.

Directions

By Car: From Geneva or Turin, take the A40 motorway to Chamonix or Courmayeur, respectively. Park in one of the designated parking areas in the town and proceed to the trailhead by foot or public transport. **By Train**: Direct trains run from Geneva or Turin to Chamonix or Courmayeur, with a travel time of approximately 1 to 2 hours. From the train station, follow signs to the Tour du Mont Blanc trailhead.

Recommended Hiking Guide Company

For those seeking guided hikes along the Tour du Mont Blanc, consider **Alpine Treks**. They offer experienced guides who are knowledgeable about the trail and can provide support services, such as luggage transfers and accommodation bookings, to enhance your hiking experience.

The Bernese Oberland Traverse

The Bernese Oberland Traverse is a scenic hiking trail that traverses the breathtaking landscapes of the Bernese Oberland region in Switzerland. This picturesque trek offers hikers the opportunity to explore stunning alpine scenery, pristine lakes, and towering peaks as they journey through the heart of the Swiss Alps. The Bernese Oberland Traverse has a variety of natural wonders, including crystal-clear mountain lakes, lush meadows, and dramatic glaciers. Keep an eye out for alpine wildlife such as ibex, chamois, and golden eagles, as well as rare plant species that thrive in the high-altitude environment. Along the way, you'll also discover charming mountain huts, traditional alpine farms, and historic villages that offer insight into the region's rich cultural heritage.

Altitude, Length, and Difficulty Level

The Bernese Oberland Traverse covers a distance of approximately 100 kilometers (62 miles) and typically takes between 5 to 7 days to complete, depending on the specific route and itinerary chosen. The trail ascends and descends over mountain passes and cols, with elevations ranging from 600 meters (1,968 feet) to over 2,000 meters (6,560 feet) above sea level. The difficulty level varies from moderate to strenuous, with long days of hiking and challenging terrain.

Route, Distance, Time, and Grade

The Bernese Oberland Traverse follows a well-marked route that winds its way through the Bernese Oberland region, passing through charming alpine villages and remote mountain valleys. A typical day on the trail may cover a distance of 15 to 20 kilometers (9 to 12 miles) and take between 6 to 8 hours to complete, including breaks and rest stops. The terrain varies from gentle forest paths to rocky mountain trails, with sections of steep ascents and descents.

Hiking Regulations

Pets are generally allowed on the Bernese Oberland Traverse but should be kept on a leash and under control at all times, especially in areas with livestock or wildlife. Hikers are also encouraged to follow Leave No Trace principles, respecting the natural environment and minimizing their impact on the trails.

Closest Accommodation: (Hotel Jungfrau Lodge: Dorfstrasse 49, 3818 Grindelwald. Situated in the heart of Grindelwald, this cozy hotel offers comfortable rooms and stunning views of the Eiger, making it an ideal base for exploring the region.) (**Mountain Hostel Grindelwald**: Hinter der Kirche 1, 3818 Grindelwald. Located in the center of Grindelwald, this budget-friendly hostel provides basic accommodation and a welcoming atmosphere for hikers and travelers.)

Closest Places to Eat: (Restaurant Belvedere: Terrassenweg 14, 3818 Grindelwald. This charming restaurant offers traditional Swiss cuisine with panoramic views of the surrounding mountains, providing a delightful dining experience after a day on the trail.) (**Restaurant Chalet Grindelwald**: Gehrenweg 15, 3818 Grindelwald. Nestled in a rustic chalet setting, this cozy restaurant serves hearty alpine dishes and local specialties, perfect for refueling and relaxing after a day of hiking.)

Logistics Upon Arrival

Parking is available in Grindelwald at designated parking areas, with daily rates typically ranging from CHF 10 to CHF 20. Alternatively, visitors can reach Grindelwald by train from major cities like Zurich and Bern, with regular services running throughout the day.

Location

The Bernese Oberland Traverse is located in the Bernese Oberland region of Switzerland, encompassing picturesque towns and villages such as Grindelwald, Wengen, and Mürren. The trail offers breathtaking views of iconic Swiss landmarks such as the Eiger, Mönch, and Jungfrau mountains.

Directions

By Car: From Zurich or Bern, take the A8 motorway to Interlaken, then follow signs for Grindelwald or Lauterbrunnen, depending on your chosen starting point for the hike. Park in one of the designated parking areas in the town and proceed to the trailhead by foot or public transport.

By Train: Direct trains run from Zurich or Bern to Interlaken, where you can transfer to regional trains or buses bound for Grindelwald or Lauterbrunnen. From there, follow signs to the Bernese Oberland Traverse trailhead.

The Via Bernina

The Via Bernina is a historic and scenic hiking trail that traverses the Swiss Alps, offering breathtaking views of alpine landscapes, charming villages, and ancient landmarks. This ancient route follows the path of the Bernina railway line, passing through tunnels, over viaducts, and alongside crystal-clear mountain streams. Highlights of the Via Bernina include the iconic Landwasser Viaduct, the picturesque Morteratsch Glacier, and the historic town of Poschiavo. Along the way, hikers can expect to encounter a variety of flora and fauna, including alpine wildflowers, chamois, and marmots.

Location of Trail

The Via Bernina runs through the canton of Graubünden in eastern Switzerland, connecting the towns of Thusis and Tirano. The trail is easily accessible from major cities like Zurich and Milan, making it a popular destination for hikers and outdoor enthusiasts.

Altitude, Length, and Difficulty Level

The trail varies in altitude, ranging from approximately 585 meters (1,919 feet) in Thusis to 1,230 meters (4,035 feet) in Tirano. The total length of the Via Bernina is approximately 135 kilometers (84 miles), with several stages ranging from easy to moderate in difficulty.

Route, Distance, Time, and Grade

The Via Bernina is divided into multiple stages, each offering its unique attractions and challenges. A typical stage covers a distance of 10 to 20 kilometers (6 to 12 miles) and takes between 3 to 6 hours to complete, depending on the pace of the hiker and the terrain. The trail is generally well-marked and maintained, with a variety of surfaces ranging from paved paths to rugged mountain trails.

Hiking Regulations

Pets are generally allowed on the Via Bernina but should be kept on a leash, especially in areas with wildlife or grazing livestock. Hikers are also reminded to respect the natural environment and adhere to local regulations regarding waste disposal and environmental protection.

Closest Accommodation: (Hotel Post: Plaza Nova 2, 7500 St. Moritz. This historic hotel is situated in the center of St. Moritz, offering comfortable rooms and easy access to the trailhead.), **(Hotel La Romantica**: Via Ronco 39, 7742 Poschiavo. Situated in the picturesque town of Poschiavo, this charming hotel provides cozy accommodation and stunning views of the surrounding mountains.)

Closest Places to Eat: (Restaurant Albergo Ristorante Bernina: Via Principale 21, 7742 Poschiavo. This cozy restaurant serves delicious Italian and Swiss cuisine, with indoor and outdoor seating options.) **(Gasthaus Alte Post**: Alte Berninastrasse 2, 7503 Samedan. Located near the town of Samedan, this traditional inn offers hearty mountain dishes and a warm atmosphere.)

Logistics Upon Arrival

Parking is available in the towns along the Via Bernina, with hourly rates typically ranging from CHF 1 to CHF 3. The trail is accessible by train from major cities like Zurich and Milan, with regular services running to stations along the route.

Directions

By Car: From Zurich, take the A13 motorway towards Thusis. Follow signs for the Via Bernina and park in one of the designated parking areas in Thusis or Tirano.

By Train: Direct trains run from Zurich to Thusis and Milan to Tirano, with a travel time of approximately 2 to 3 hours. From Thusis or Tirano, take the local train to stations along the Via Bernina.

Recommended Hiking Guide Company

For those looking for guided hikes along the Via Bernina, consider **Swiss Alpine Adventures**.

The Jura Crest Trail

The Jura Crest Trail winds its way along the ridgeline of the Jura Mountains, offering hikers breathtaking views of rolling hills, deep valleys, and lush forests. This picturesque trail showcases the natural beauty and rich biodiversity of the region, making it a favorite among nature lovers and outdoor enthusiasts. As you hike the Jura Crest Trail, you'll encounter a variety of flora and fauna unique to the Jura Mountains. Keep an eye out for rare orchids, colorful butterflies, and elusive red deer as you traverse through dense forests and open meadows. Along the way, you'll also discover charming villages, ancient ruins, and historical landmarks that offer insight into the region's cultural heritage.

Location of Trail

The Jura Crest Trail stretches along the border between Switzerland and France, running from Dielsdorf in the north to Nyon in the south. The trailhead is easily accessible from major cities like Zurich and Geneva, making it a convenient destination for day hikes or multi-day treks.

Altitude, Length, and Difficulty Level

The trail varies in altitude, with elevations ranging from approximately 400 meters (1,312 feet) to 1,672 meters (5,486 feet) at its highest point. The total length of the Jura Crest Trail is approximately 310 kilometers (193 miles), offering a variety of routes suitable for hikers of all skill levels. While some sections may be challenging, the trail is generally well-marked and maintained, making it accessible to both beginners and experienced hikers.

Route, Distance, Time, and Grade

The Jura Crest Trail is divided into multiple stages, each covering a distance of 10 to 20 kilometers (6 to 12 miles) and taking between 4 to 8 hours to complete, depending on the terrain and pace of the hiker. The trail features a mix of gentle ascents, gradual descents, and flat sections, with occasional rocky or muddy patches. Hikers can expect to encounter a variety of surfaces, including dirt paths, gravel tracks, and paved roads.

Hiking Regulations

While pets are generally allowed on the Jura Crest Trail, it's important to keep them on a leash and under control at all times, especially in areas with livestock or wildlife. Hikers are also encouraged to follow Leave No Trace principles, respecting the natural environment and minimizing their impact on the trails.

Closest Accommodation: (Hôtel de la Couronne: Rue de l'Hôtel de Ville 16, 2900 Porrentruy. This charming hotel is located near the town of Porrentruy, offering comfortable rooms and easy access to the trailhead.) (**Auberge de la Gare**: Rue de la Gare 1, 1347 Le Sentier. Situated in the village of Le Sentier, this cozy inn provides affordable accommodation and stunning views of the surrounding countryside.)

Closest Places to Eat: (Restaurant La Bonne Auberge: Rue de la Promenade 21, 2900 Porrentruy. This traditional restaurant serves hearty Swiss cuisine and is a popular spot for locals and visitors alike.)

(**Auberge du Prévoux**: Le Prévoux 1, 1345 Le Lieu. Located near the village of Le Lieu, this rustic inn offers delicious regional dishes and a warm atmosphere.)

Logistics Upon Arrival

Parking is available in Porrentruy and Le Sentier at designated areas, with hourly rates typically ranging from CHF 1 to CHF 3. The trailheads can be reached by car or public transport from nearby towns and cities.

Directions

By Car: From Zurich or Geneva, take the A1 motorway to Yverdon-les-Bains, then follow signs for the Jura Crest Trail. Park in one of the designated parking areas in Porrentruy or Le Sentier and proceed to the trailhead by foot or public transport. **By Train**: Direct trains run from Zurich or Geneva to Yverdon-les-Bains, where you can transfer to regional trains or buses bound for Porrentruy or Le Sentier.

From there, follow signs to the Jura Crest Trail. For those seeking guided hikes along the Jura Crest Trail, consider **Jura Adventures**.

The Jungfrau Panorama Trail

The Jungfrau Panorama Trail is a stunning alpine hike that offers unparalleled views of the famous Jungfrau massif and surrounding peaks. This scenic route winds its way through lush meadows, past sparkling mountain streams, and beneath towering glaciers, providing hikers with a true taste of Swiss mountain beauty. Highlights of the Jungfrau Panorama Trail include breathtaking vistas of the Eiger, Monch, and Jungfrau peaks, as well as close-up views of the UNESCO-listed Aletsch Glacier, the longest glacier in the Alps. Along the way, hikers may also encounter alpine wildlife such as ibex, chamois, and marmots, as well as a variety of alpine flora including edelweiss and gentian.

Location of Trail

The Jungfrau Panorama Trail is located in the Bernese Oberland region of Switzerland, near the towns of Grindelwald, Wengen, and Lauterbrunnen. The trailhead can be easily accessed by public transport from major cities like Bern and Zurich, making it a popular destination for hikers from all over the world.

Altitude, Length, and Difficulty Level

The trail varies in altitude, with starting points typically around 1,000 meters (3,280 feet) above sea level and reaching heights of up to 2,000 meters (6,560 feet) or more. The total length of the Jungfrau Panorama Trail depends on the specific route chosen, but most sections are between 10 to 15 kilometers (6 to 9 miles) long. The difficulty level ranges from easy to moderate, with well-marked paths and occasional steep sections.

Route, Distance, Time, and Grade

The Jungfrau Panorama Trail follows a series of interconnected paths and mountain tracks, offering hikers a variety of route options depending on their preferences and fitness levels. A typical section of the trail may take between 3 to 5 hours to complete, including time for breaks and photo stops. The terrain is generally well-maintained and suitable for hikers of all abilities, although some sections may be rocky or steep.

Hiking Regulations

Pets are generally allowed on the Jungfrau Panorama Trail but should be kept on a leash, especially in areas with grazing livestock or sensitive wildlife habitats. Hikers are also reminded to stay on designated paths and respect any posted signs or guidelines to minimize their impact on the fragile alpine ecosystem.

Closest Accommodation: (Hotel Bellevue des Alpes: Dorfstrasse 58, 3818 Grindelwald. This historic hotel offers comfortable rooms and stunning views of the Eiger, Monch, and Jungfrau peaks, making it an ideal base for exploring the area.)

(**Hotel Edelweiss**: Dorfstrasse 5, 3823 Wengen. Situated in the car-free village of Wengen, this cozy hotel provides a peaceful retreat after a day of hiking, with easy access to the Jungfrau Panorama Trail.)

Closest Places to Eat: (Restaurant Eigernordwand: Eigernordwand, 3818 Grindelwald. This mountain restaurant offers hearty Swiss cuisine and panoramic views of the surrounding peaks, perfect for refueling after a day on the trail.)

(**Restaurant Männlichen**: Männlichen, 3823 Wengen. Located at the Männlichen gondola station, this restaurant serves a variety of alpine dishes and refreshments, with outdoor seating overlooking the Jungfrau massif.)

Logistics Upon Arrival

Parking is available in the towns of Grindelwald, Wengen, and Lauterbrunnen, with hourly rates typically ranging from CHF 1 to CHF 3. The trailheads can be reached by train or cable car from these towns, with regular services running throughout the day.

Directions

By Car: From Bern or Zurich, take the A8 motorway to Interlaken, then follow signs for Grindelwald, Wengen, or Lauterbrunnen, depending on your chosen starting point for the hike. Park in one of the designated parking areas in the town and proceed to the trailhead by foot or public transport. **By Train**: Direct trains run from Bern or Zurich to Interlaken, where you can transfer to regional trains or cable cars bound for

Grindelwald, Wengen, or Lauterbrunnen. From there, follow signs to the Jungfrau Panorama Trail.

Recommended Hiking Guide Company

 Alpine Adventures Switzerland. They offer experienced guides who can lead you on customized tours tailored to your interests and fitness level.

The Zermatt Glacier Trail

The Zermatt Glacier Trail is an epic alpine adventure that takes hikers on a journey through the heart of the Swiss Alps, offering unrivaled views of majestic peaks, vast glaciers, and pristine alpine landscapes. This challenging route traverses high mountain passes, rugged terrain, and icy slopes, providing an unforgettable experience for experienced hikers and mountaineers. Highlights of the Zermatt Glacier Trail include close-up views of iconic peaks such as the Matterhorn, Monte Rosa, and Weisshorn, as well as encounters with glaciers such as the Gorner Glacier and the Theodul Glacier. Along the way, hikers may also encounter alpine wildlife such as ibex, chamois, and mountain goats, as well as a variety of alpine flora including alpine roses and gentian.

Location of Trail

The Zermatt Glacier Trail is located in the canton of Valais in southwestern Switzerland, near the famous mountain resort town of Zermatt. The trailhead can be easily accessed by public transport from major cities like Zurich and Geneva, making it a popular destination for hikers and mountaineers from all over the world.

Altitude, Length, and Difficulty Level

The trail varies in altitude, with starting points typically around 1,600 meters (5,250 feet) above sea level and reaching heights of up to 3,000 meters (9,840 feet) or more. The total length of the Zermatt Glacier Trail is approximately 25 kilometers (15.5 miles), with several stages ranging from moderate to strenuous in difficulty.

Route, Distance, Time, and Grade

The Zermatt Glacier Trail follows a challenging route through high alpine terrain, with steep ascents, rocky paths, and icy sections. A typical stage of the trail may cover a distance of 10 to 15 kilometers (6 to 9 miles) and take between 6 to 8 hours to complete, depending on the pace of the hiker and the conditions. The terrain is rugged and exposed, requiring a good level of fitness and mountain hiking experience.

Hiking Regulations

Due to the challenging nature of the Zermatt Glacier Trail, it is recommended for experienced hikers and mountaineers only. Pets are generally not allowed on this trail due to the hazardous terrain and potential dangers posed by glaciers and crevasses. Hikers are advised to check local weather and trail conditions before embarking on the hike and to be prepared for changing conditions at high altitudes.

Closest Accommodation: (Hotel Monte Rosa: Bahnhofstrasse 80, 3920 Zermatt. Located in the heart of Zermatt, this historic hotel offers comfortable rooms and stunning views of the Matterhorn, making it an ideal base for exploring the area.)

(Riffelhaus 1853: Riffelberg, 3920 Zermatt. Situated at an altitude of 2,582 meters (8,471 feet), this mountain hotel provides cozy accommodation and direct access to the trailhead, allowing hikers to start their adventure right from the doorstep.)

Closest Places to Eat: (Restaurant Chez Vrony: Findeln, 3920 Zermatt. This rustic mountain restaurant serves traditional Swiss cuisine and homemade specialties, with panoramic views of the surrounding peaks.)

(Restaurant Schwarzsee: Schwarzsee, 3920 Zermatt. Located near the Schwarzsee gondola station, this restaurant offers a variety of alpine dishes and refreshments, perfect for refueling after a day on the trail.)

Logistics Upon Arrival

Parking is available in Zermatt at designated parking areas, with hourly rates typically ranging from CHF 1 to CHF 3. Alternatively, visitors can reach Zermatt by train from major cities like Zurich and Geneva, with regular services running throughout the day. From Zermatt, hikers can take the Gornergrat Railway or the Schwarzsee cable car to access the trailhead.

Directions

By Car: From Zurich or Geneva, take the A9 motorway to Visp, then follow the signs for Zermatt. Park in one of the designated parking areas in Zermatt and proceed to the Gornergrat Railway or the Schwarzsee cable car station to access the trailhead. **By Train**: Direct trains run from Zurich or Geneva to Visp, where you can transfer to the Matterhorn Gotthard Bahn for the final leg of the journey to Zermatt. From Zermatt, take the Gornergrat Railway or the Schwarzsee cable car to reach the trailhead.

Recommended Hiking Guide Company

Alpin Center Zermatt. They offer experienced guides who can lead you on challenging mountain adventures, including the Zermatt Glacier Trail. Contact them via their website or visit their office in Zermatt for more information.

The Grisons Panorama Trail

The Grisons Panorama Trail is a spectacular hiking route that winds its way through the breathtaking landscapes of the Swiss canton of Graubünden, offering panoramic views of snow-capped peaks, crystal-clear lakes, and picturesque alpine villages. This scenic trail showcases the natural beauty and cultural heritage of the region, passing through lush forests, rolling meadows, and rugged mountain passes.

Highlights of the Grisons Panorama Trail include stunning vistas of the Piz Bernina, the highest peak in the Eastern Alps, as well as encounters with local wildlife such as red deer, chamois, and golden eagles. Along the way, hikers can explore historic villages, visit traditional alpine farms, and learn about the unique customs and traditions of the Graubünden region.

Location of Trail

The Grisons Panorama Trail spans the canton of Graubünden in eastern Switzerland, covering a diverse range of landscapes and ecosystems. The trailhead can be easily accessed by public transport from major cities like Zurich and Milan, making it a popular destination for hikers and nature lovers.

Altitude, Length, and Difficulty Level

The trail varies in altitude, with starting points typically between 1,000 to 1,500 meters (3,280 to 4,920 feet) above sea level and reaching heights of up to 2,500 meters (8,200 feet) or more. The total length of the Grisons Panorama Trail is approximately 150 kilometers (93 miles), with multiple stages ranging from easy to moderate in difficulty.

Outlining Route, Distance, Time, and Grade

The Grisons Panorama Trail follows a well-marked route through some of the most scenic areas of Graubünden, with gentle gradients and moderate ascents and descents. A typical stage of the trail may cover a distance of 10 to 20 kilometers (6 to 12 miles) and take between 4 to 6 hours to complete, depending on the pace of the hiker and the terrain.

The trail is suitable for hikers of all abilities, with options for shorter or longer routes depending on preferences.

Hiking Regulations

Pets are generally allowed on the Grisons Panorama Trail but should be kept on a leash, especially in areas with grazing livestock or sensitive wildlife habitats. Hikers are also reminded to stay on designated paths and respect any posted signs or guidelines to minimize their impact on the natural environment.

Closest Accommodation: (Hotel Kulm: Via Veglia 1, 7500 St. Moritz. Located in the heart of St. Moritz, this luxury hotel offers elegant rooms and world-class amenities, making it an ideal base for exploring the Graubünden region.)

(Hotel La Veduta: Via Tignons 6, 7742 Poschiavo. Situated in the charming village of Poschiavo, this cozy hotel provides comfortable accommodation and easy access to the trailhead.)

Closest Places to Eat

(Restaurant Chesa Veglia: Via Veglia 18, 7500 St. Moritz. This historic restaurant serves gourmet Swiss cuisine in a cozy Alpine setting, with options for indoor and outdoor dining.)

(Ristorante La Posta: Via Principale 51, 7742 Poschiavo. Located in the heart of Poschiavo, this family-run restaurant offers traditional Italian dishes and local specialties, with a warm and welcoming atmosphere.)

Logistics Upon Arrival

Parking is available in St. Moritz and Poschiavo at designated parking areas, with hourly rates typically ranging from CHF 1 to CHF 3. Alternatively, visitors can reach St. Moritz and Poschiavo by train from major cities like Zurich and Milan, with regular services running throughout the day. From there, hikers can access the trailhead by foot or public transport.

Directions

By Car: From Zurich or Milan, take the A13 motorway towards St. Moritz or Poschiavo, respectively. Follow signs for the town center and park in one of the designated parking areas. From there, proceed to the trailhead by foot or public transport. **By Train**: Direct trains run from Zurich to St. Moritz and Milan to Poschiavo, with a travel time of approximately 3 to 4 hours. From St. Moritz or Poschiavo, hikers can take local buses or taxis to reach the trailhead.

Recommended Hiking Guide Company

Consider **Alpine Adventures Graubünden**. They offer experienced guides who are familiar with the trails and terrain of the area, providing customized tours and excursions for hikers of all levels. Contact them via their website or visit their office in St. Moritz for more information.

The Susten Pass Trail

The Susten Pass Trail offers a stunning mix of alpine scenery, challenging terrain, and rich history. This trail, located in the Swiss Alps, climbs to an altitude of 2,264 meters, stretching over 6.5 kilometers. It's considered moderately difficult, making it suitable for hikers with a good fitness level.

On this trail, hikers are treated to an array of beautiful alpine flora, including edelweiss and alpine roses. Wildlife sightings might include ibexes and marmots, which add a special charm to the journey. Historically, the Susten Pass has been a vital route linking the Reuss and Aare valleys, and remnants of old trading paths can still be seen.

The hike typically takes about 3 to 4 hours, with a steady incline and some rocky sections that require careful footing. Along the way, you'll enjoy breathtaking views of glaciers and the imposing peaks of the Urner Alps.

As for hiking regulations, dogs are allowed on the Susten Pass Trail, provided they are on a leash. It's essential to stick to the marked paths to protect the delicate alpine environment.

For accommodations, consider staying at Hotel Steingletscher, Sustenstrasse 2, 3863 Gadmen, or Hotel Tiefenbach, Sustenpass, 6487 Wassen. Both offer comfortable lodgings with easy access to the trailhead.

After your hike, enjoy a meal at the Restaurant Steingletscher, located at the start of the trail, or Gasthaus Göscheneralp at Göscheneralpstrasse, 6487 Göschenen.

Parking is available at the Steingletscher parking lot, with a small fee of CHF 5 per day. The Susten Pass is accessible from the town of Innertkirchen via Route 11. GPS coordinates for the trailhead are 46.7369° N, 8.4363° E.

For a guided experience, contact Alpine Hiking.ch, Hauptstrasse 15, 3863 Gadmen. They offer knowledgeable guides familiar with the Susten Pass Trail and can enhance your hiking experience with local insights.

The Titlis Cliff Walk

The Titlis Cliff Walk is an exhilarating trail offering a unique alpine adventure. Located at an altitude of 3,041 meters, this 1-kilometer walk is relatively short but provides an adrenaline rush with its suspension bridge spanning a dizzying height over the Titlis glacier.

The trail is fairly easy and suitable for most hikers, taking about 30 minutes to complete. You'll find yourself surrounded by stunning snow-covered peaks and deep glacier crevasses. The views are panoramic, stretching across the Bernese Alps and even reaching as far as the Black Forest in Germany on clear days.

Since this is a high-altitude trail, proper warm clothing and sturdy footwear are essential. Pets are not allowed on the Titlis Cliff Walk due to safety concerns.

Accommodation options include the Berghotel Trübsee, Trübsee, 6390 Engelberg, and Hotel Terrace, Terracestrasse 33, 6390 Engelberg. Both offer cozy stays with beautiful alpine views.

For dining, the Panorama Restaurant Titlis, located at the top of Mount Titlis, offers delicious meals with a view. Alternatively, the Titlis Mountain Restaurant at the Trübsee midway station is a great option.

Parking is available at the Engelberg-Titlis parking lot, costing CHF 5 per day. Engelberg is the closest town, and the trail is accessible via the Titlis Rotair cable car from Engelberg. The GPS coordinates for the trail are 46.7729° N and 8.4350° E.

For guided tours, contact Titlis Tours, Gerschnistrasse 12, 6390 Engelberg, which offers professional guides for the Titlis Cliff Walk.

The Matterhorn Glacier Trail

The Matterhorn Glacier Trail is a spectacular hike offering close-up views of the iconic Matterhorn. Starting at an altitude of 2,939 meters, this 6.5-kilometer trail is considered moderately challenging, with a duration of about 2 to 3 hours.

This trail winds through a landscape of moraines, glacial streams, and ice formations, with informative panels about the geology and glaciology of the region. You might encounter marmots and chamois, adding a touch of wildlife to the trek.

Due to the high altitude and uneven terrain, hikers should be well-prepared with appropriate gear. Pets are allowed on the trail if kept on a leash.

Stay at Hotel Schwarzsee, Schwarzsee, 3920 Zermatt, or Hotel Alpenrose, Riedweg 96, 3920 Zermatt, both offering excellent accommodations with easy access to the trail.

Dine at Restaurant Schwarzsee, near the trailhead, or the Restaurant Stafelalp, Stafelalp, 3920 Zermatt, for a hearty meal after your hike.

Parking is available in Täsch, with a shuttle service to Zermatt. The trail starts from the Trockener Steg station, reachable via cable car from Zermatt. GPS coordinates are 45.9763° N, 7.6586° E.

For guided hikes, contact Zermatters, Bahnhofstrasse 58, 3920 Zermatt, offering expert guides for the Matterhorn Glacier Trail.

The Bannalp Circular Trail

The Bannalp Circular Trail is a delightful loop offering serene alpine scenery. Situated at an altitude of 1,600 meters, this 8-kilometer trail is moderately difficult, taking about 3 to 4 hours to complete.

The trail traverses lush meadows filled with wildflowers and passes by tranquil alpine lakes. You might spot ibex and golden eagles during your hike. Historical markers along the way provide insights into the region's past.

Dogs are welcome on the trail but must be kept on a leash to protect the wildlife.

For accommodations, try Gasthaus Urnerstaffel, Urnerstaffel, 6375 Bannalp, or Berggasthaus Bannalpsee, Bannalpsee, 6375 Wolfenschiessen, both offering a rustic alpine experience.

Enjoy meals at the Bergrestaurant Bannalp, Bannalp, 6375 Wolfenschiessen, or the Gasthaus Urnerstaffel for local cuisine.

Parking is available at the Fellboden parking lot, costing CHF 5 per day. The trailhead is accessible from Wolfenschiessen, with a cable car ride from Fellboden. GPS coordinates are 46.8783° N, 8.3861° E.

For guided tours, contact Swiss Hike Guide, Dorfstrasse 27, 6375 Wolfenschiessen, offering personalized hiking experiences in Bannalp.

The Pigne d'Arolla Trail

The Pigne d'Arolla Trail is a challenging hike reserved for experienced hikers. Rising to an altitude of 3,796 meters, this 12-kilometer trail offers breathtaking views and takes about 8 to 10 hours to complete.

This high-altitude trail traverses glaciated terrain, with stunning views of the Mont Collon and the Arolla glaciers. The trail is rich in alpine flora and fauna, including sightings of chamois and alpine ibex.

Given its difficulty and altitude, proper gear, including crampons and ice axes, is necessary. Pets are not recommended due to the challenging nature of the trail.

Stay at Hotel du Pigne, Route de l'eglise, 1986 Arolla, or Grand Hotel Kurhaus, Route des Arolles, 1986 Arolla, both providing comfortable lodging close to the trailhead.

For dining, visit Restaurant du Pigne, Route de l'eglise, 1986 Arolla, or La Gouille Restaurant, La Gouille, 1986 Arolla.

Parking is available at the Arolla Village parking lot, free of charge. The trailhead starts at the Arolla village. GPS coordinates are 46.0230° N, 7.4927° E.

For a guided hike, contact Alpine Guides Arolla, Chemin de l'École 8, 1986 Arolla, specializing in high-altitude treks like the Pigne d'Arolla.

The Wildstrubel Panorama Trail

The Wildstrubel Panorama Trail offers a captivating hike through the scenic landscapes of the Bernese Alps. The trail starts at an altitude of 2,400 meters and stretches for 15 kilometers, presenting a moderately challenging experience for hikers. The path winds through lush alpine meadows, dotted with a variety of wildflowers such as gentians and edelweiss, and offers frequent encounters with marmots and chamois.

The trail begins at the Gemmi Pass, accessible by a cable car from Leukerbad. The hike takes around 5 to 6 hours, with gradual ascents and descents providing stunning panoramic views of the Wildstrubel massif and the surrounding peaks.

Hikers should be prepared for varying weather conditions and bring appropriate gear. Pets are allowed but must be kept on a leash to protect the local wildlife. Stick to the marked paths to preserve the natural environment.

For a comfortable stay, consider Hotel Alfa Soleil at 3718 Kandersteg or the Hotel Waldhaus at Dorfstrasse 6, 3954 Leukerbad. Both offer cozy accommodations with easy access to the trail.

After your hike, enjoy a meal at the Restaurant Gemmi Lodge, located at the trailhead, or the Panorama Restaurant at the summit of the Gemmi Pass.

Parking is available at the Leukerbad cable car station, with a daily fee of CHF 5. The trailhead is located at Gemmi Pass, which is reachable by cable car. GPS coordinates for the trailhead are 46.3790° N, 7.6211° E.

For guided hikes, contact Wildstrubel Trekking, located at Dorfstrasse 8, 3954 Leukerbad. They offer experienced guides who can enrich your hiking experience with local knowledge.

The Brienzergrat Ridge Trail

The Brienzergrat Ridge Trail is a spectacular hike along one of the most scenic ridges in Switzerland. Starting at an altitude of 2,350 meters, this 20-kilometer trail is challenging and best suited for experienced hikers. The hike takes approximately 8 to 10 hours, offering stunning views of Lake Brienz and the surrounding peaks.

This ridge walk is a botanist's delight, with an abundance of alpine flora, including orchids and mountain asters. Keep an eye out for ibex and golden eagles soaring above. The trail also passes several historical sites, including old shepherd huts and boundary markers dating back centuries.

Due to the trail's difficulty and exposed sections, hikers should be well-prepared with proper gear. Pets are not recommended on this trail due to its challenging nature.

For accommodation, stay at the Grandhotel Giessbach, Axalpstrasse, 3855 Brienz, or the Hotel Brienzerburli, Hauptstrasse 11, 3855 Brienz. Both provide excellent lodging options close to the trail.

Dine at the Restaurant Rothorn Kulm, located at the Brienzer Rothorn summit, or the Bramisegg Restaurant, located midway along the trail.

Parking is available at the Brienz Rothorn Bahn station, costing CHF 5 per day. The trailhead is accessible by taking the Brienz Rothorn Bahn train to the summit station. GPS coordinates for the trailhead are 46.7767° N, 8.0666° E.

For guided tours, contact Brienz Guides, Hauptstrasse 120, 3855 Brienz. They specialize in guided hikes along the Brienzergrat Ridge.

The Diablerets Glacier Trail

The Diablerets Glacier Trail offers an incredible hike across a majestic glacier. Starting at an altitude of 3,000 meters, this 12-kilometer trail is moderately difficult and takes about 5 to 6 hours to complete. The trail features stunning glacial landscapes, ice formations, and panoramic views of the Alps.

Along the way, hikers will encounter a variety of alpine plants and possibly see wildlife such as snow hares and ptarmigans. Historical points of interest include the old glacier cabins used by early mountaineers.

Given the glacial environment, hikers need proper gear, including crampons and warm clothing. Pets are not allowed on the glacier for safety reasons.

Stay at the Hotel Les Sources, Chemin du Vernex 9, 1865 Les Diablerets, or the Eurotel Victoria Les Diablerets, Chemin du Vernex 3, 1865 Les Diablerets. Both offer excellent accommodations near the trailhead.

After your hike, enjoy a meal at the Glacier 3000 Restaurant at the trailhead or Auberge de la Poste, Rue de la Gare, 1865 Les Diablerets.

Parking is available at the Glacier 3000 cable car station, with a fee of CHF 5 per day. The trailhead is accessible via the Glacier 3000 cable car. GPS coordinates for the trailhead are 46.3408° N, 7.2081° E.

For guided hikes, contact Diablerets Mountain Guides, Route du Pillon 253, 1865 Les Diablerets. They offer professional guides for the Diablerets Glacier Trail.

The Pilatus Summit Trail

The Pilatus Summit Trail offers a rewarding hike to the summit of Mount Pilatus. Starting at an altitude of 1,400 meters and rising to 2,128 meters, this 7-kilometer trail is moderately difficult and takes about 3 to 4 hours to complete. The trail features a mix of forested paths, rocky climbs, and panoramic views over Lake Lucerne and the surrounding mountains.

The trail is home to various plants, including alpine roses and gentians, and wildlife such as chamois and marmots. Historical highlights include the medieval Pilatus Kulm and legends associated with the mountain.

Hikers should be prepared for varying weather conditions and bring appropriate gear. Pets are allowed on the trail if kept on a leash.

Stay at the Hotel Pilatus-Kulm, Pilatus, 6010 Kriens, or the Bellevue Hotel, Pilatus, 6010 Kriens. Both offer excellent accommodations at the summit.

After your hike, enjoy a meal at the Pilatus-Kulm Restaurant or the Bellevue Restaurant, both offering local cuisine with stunning views.

Parking is available at the Pilatusbahn station in Kriens, costing CHF 5 per day. The trailhead is accessible by taking the Pilatusbahn cable car to Fräkmüntegg. GPS coordinates for the trailhead are 46.9784° N, 8.2535° E.

For guided hikes, contact Pilatus Guides, Schlossberg 1, 6010 Kriens. They provide experienced guides for the Pilatus Summit Trail.

Conclusion

In conclusion, hiking in Switzerland offers an unparalleled opportunity to connect with nature, explore stunning landscapes, and embark on unforgettable adventures. From towering mountain peaks to pristine alpine meadows, Switzerland's diverse terrain provides endless opportunities for outdoor enthusiasts of all ages and skill levels.

Throughout your hiking journey in Switzerland, you'll discover a wealth of natural wonders, from cascading waterfalls and turquoise lakes to majestic glaciers and ancient forests. Each trail offers its unique charms and challenges, inviting you to immerse yourself in the beauty and tranquility of the Swiss Alps.

Whether you're seeking a stroll along gentle valley paths or a challenging ascent to a lofty summit, Switzerland has a trail to suit every preference and ability. Along the way, you'll encounter a rich tapestry of flora and fauna, with opportunities to spot rare alpine flowers, elusive wildlife, and vibrant birdlife.

But hiking in Switzerland is not just about the destination—it's about the journey itself. As you traverse winding mountain trails, navigate rocky ridges, and breathe in the crisp alpine air, you'll experience a sense of freedom and exhilaration like no other. Each step brings you closer to nature, allowing you to leave behind the stresses of daily life and reconnect with the world around you.

As you reflect on your hiking adventures in Switzerland, take pride in the memories you've created, the challenges you've overcome, and the bonds you've forged with fellow hikers and loved ones. Remember to cherish these moments, and let them inspire you to seek out new trails, new experiences, and new horizons in the future.

In the end, hiking in Switzerland is more than just a physical activity—it's a journey of the heart, a celebration of the beauty and majesty of the natural world, and a reminder of the joys of exploration and discovery. So lace up your boots, pack your backpack, and set out on the trail with confidence, knowing that the wonders of Switzerland await you at every turn.

Appendices

Glossary of Hiking Terms

- *Trailhead: The begining of a hiking trail.*
- *Switchback: A zigzagging trail that ascends or descends a steep slope.*
- *Cairn: A pack of rocks used as a trail marker.*
- *Summit: The highest point of a mountain or peak.*
- *Basecamp: A central campsite used as a starting point for hiking expeditions.*
- *Backpacking: Hiking and camping overnight with a backpack containing necessary gear and supplies.*
- *Trekking poles: Adjustable poles used for stability and balance while hiking.*
- *Scrambling: Climbing steep rock faces or boulders using hands and feet.*
- *Thru-hike: Hiking an entire long-distance trail from start to finish in one continuous journey.*
- *Water filtration: Process of purifying water from natural sources for safe consumption.*
- *Shelter: A tent or other protective structure used for overnight camping.*
- *Bear canister: A portable container used to store food and other scented items to prevent attracting bears.*
- *Trail etiquette: Rules and practices for courteous behavior on hiking trails.*

- *Leave No Trace: Principles for minimizing environmental impact while hiking and camping.*
- *Blister: A painful swelling caused by friction between the skin and footwear.*
- *GPS: Global Positioning System, a satellite-based navigation system used for determining location on a trail.*
- *Altitude sickness: Symptoms such as headache, nausea, and fatigue caused by exposure to high altitudes.*
- *Map and compass: Tools used for navigation while hiking in remote areas.*
- *Wilderness permit: Authorization required for hiking and camping in designated wilderness areas.*
- *Bear spray: A deterrent used to deter aggressive bears during encounters.*
- *Trail mix: A snack made of dried fruits, nuts, and sometimes chocolate or granola.*
- *Ultralight: Gear and equipment designed to be lightweight for backpacking and hiking.*
- *Waterproof: Resistant to water penetration, often used to describe clothing, footwear, and gear.*
- *Trail register: A logbook or sign-in sheet at the trailhead for hikers to record their presence.*
- *Blazing: Markings such as paint or tape used to indicate a hiking trail.*
- *Headlamp: A hands-free light source worn on the head for hiking in low-light conditions or at night.*
- *Compass rose: Symbol on a map indicating direction, usually with north at the top.*

- *Wayfinding: Navigating and orienting oneself in unfamiliar terrain.*
- *Bear hang A method of suspending food and scented items out of reach of bears while camping.*
- *Dry bag: A waterproof bag used to protect gear and clothing from moisture.*
- *Daypack: A small backpack used for day hikes to carry essentials such as water, snacks, and a first aid kit.*
- *Bushwhacking: Hiking off-trail through dense vegetation.*
- *Map scale: Ratio used to represent distances on a map relative to actual distances on the ground.*
- *Contour lines: Lines on a topographic map indicating elevation changes and terrain features.*
- *Hiking boots: Sturdy footwear designed for hiking on rugged terrain.*
- *Hydration bladder: A reservoir worn inside a backpack for convenient access to water while hiking.*
- *Marmot: A large ground-dwelling rodent often seen in alpine regions.*
- *GPS coordinates: Specific geographic coordinates used for pinpointing locations on Earth.*
- *Wilderness area: A protected natural area where human activity is restricted to preserve its pristine condition.*
- *Hiking pole: A single pole used for stability and balance while hiking, often adjustable in length.*
- *Hiking socks: Specially designed socks with extra padding and moisture-wicking properties for hiking comfort.*

- *Puffy jacket: Lightweight insulated jacket designed to provide warmth in cold weather.*
- *Tarp: A large sheet of waterproof fabric used as a makeshift shelter or ground cover.*
- *Bivy sack: A lightweight, waterproof shelter designed to enclose a sleeping bag for minimalist camping.*
- *Microspikes: Traction devices worn over footwear to prevent slipping on icy or snowy trails.*
- *Wilderness survival: Skills and knowledge for surviving in remote wilderness environments.*
- *Leave-no-trace camping: Camping practices that minimize impact on the environment and wildlife.*
- *Dry-fit clothing: Moisture-wicking clothing designed to keep hikers dry and comfortable during physical activity.*
- *Hiking map: A topographic map showing trails, terrain features, and landmarks for navigation.*
- *Glissading: Sliding down a steep snow slope on foot or using a sitting position.*
- *Mountain lion: Large predatory feline species also known as a cougar or puma.*
- *Geocaching: Outdoor recreational activity of using GPS coordinates to locate hidden containers called geocaches.*
- *Trail running: Running or jogging on hiking trails for fitness and enjoyment.*
- *Avalanche safety: Knowledge and precautions for avoiding and surviving avalanches in mountainous terrain.*
- *Orienteering: Competitive sport or recreational activity involving navigation using a map and compass.*

- *Water crossing: Crossing a river, stream, or creek while hiking, often requiring caution and proper technique.*
- *Hypothermia: Dangerous drop in body temperature caused by exposure to cold and wet conditions.*
- *GPS watch: A wrist-mounted device with built-in GPS functionality for navigation and fitness tracking.*
- *Alpine start: Early morning departure for a hike or climb to take advantage of favorable weather conditions.*
- *Bear bell: A bell attached to clothing or backpacks to alert bears of human presence and reduce the risk of surprise encounters.*
- *Windbreaker: Lightweight outerwear designed to protect against wind while hiking.*
- *Alpenglow: Soft pink or reddish light often seen on mountain peaks just before sunrise or after sunset.*
- *Snowshoes: Footwear with a large surface area designed to distribute weight and prevent sinking in deep snow.*
- *Navigation app: Smartphone application used for GPS navigation and mapping while hiking.*
- *Topographic map: A detailed map showing elevation contours, terrain features, and geographic landmarks.*
- *Tree line: The elevation above which trees become smaller and sparse due to harsh alpine conditions.*
- *Glacial meltwater: Freshwater from melting glaciers often found in alpine lakes and streams.*
- *Scree slope: A steep slope covered with loose rock fragments, making for challenging terrain to navigate.*

- *Shelter-in-place: Emergency protocol for finding a safe location and remaining there during inclement weather or other hazards.*
- *High-altitude camping: Camping at elevations where oxygen levels are lower, requiring acclimatization and precautions.*
- *Lightning safety: Precautions and procedures for avoiding lightning strikes while hiking in thunderstorms.*
- *Rockfall: The sudden release of rocks or boulders from a cliff or mountainside, posing a hazard to hikers below.*
- *Bear-resistant food container: A sturdy container designed to prevent bears from accessing stored food and scented items.*
- *Talus field: An area of unstable rock debris often found at the base of cliffs or steep slopes.*
- *Snow bridge: A natural bridge formed by snow accumulation over a crevasse or stream, requiring caution when crossing.*
- *Wilderness medicine: First aid techniques and medical care for injuries and illnesses encountered in remote wilderness areas.*
- *Hypoxia: Lack of oxygen at high altitudes, leading to symptoms such as shortness of breath, dizziness, and fatigue. 78. Cairn hopping: Following a trail marked by a series of cairns.*
- *Hiker's high: The sense of euphoria and well-being experienced during or after a challenging hike.*
- *Frostbite: Injury to skin and tissue caused by exposure to extreme cold, particularly on exposed skin such as fingers, toes, and ears.*
- *Belaying: Technique used in climbing to secure a rope and protect a climber from falls.*
- *Tree well: A void or depression around the base of a tree filled with loose snow, posing a hazard to skiers and snowshoers.*

- *Alpine club: An organization dedicated to promoting hiking, climbing, and mountaineering in mountainous regions.*
- *Scenic overlook: A designated viewpoint offering panoramic views of surrounding landscapes.*
- *Route finding: The process of identifying and following a safe and efficient path through rugged terrain.*
- *Hiking buddy system: Practice of hiking in pairs or groups for safety and mutual support.*
- *Patagonia fleece: Lightweight, breathable fleece clothing designed for warmth and comfort during outdoor activities.*
- *Ice axe: A multipurpose tool used for self-arresting in snow and ice, as well as for cutting steps and anchors in mountaineering.*
- *Snakebite kit: A first aid kit containing supplies and instructions for treating snakebites in the wilderness.*
- *Avalanche beacon: A device used for locating buried avalanche victims by emitting and receiving radio signals.*
- *Wilderness therapy: Therapeutic programs and interventions conducted in outdoor wilderness settings to promote personal growth and healing.*
- *Ridge walk: Hiking along the narrow crest of a mountain ridge, offering expansive views on both sides.*
- *Gaiters: Protective coverings worn over shoes or boots to keep out snow, water, and debris.*
- *Frost heave: Upward swelling of soil and rock caused by the freezing and thawing of water in the ground.*
- *Glacial moraine: A deposit of rock debris carried and deposited by a glacier, forming a ridge or mound.*

- *Leave a trace: The philosophy of minimizing impact and leaving minimal evidence of human presence in the wilderness.*
- *Wilderness ranger: A trained professional responsible for managing and protecting wilderness areas and enforcing regulations.*
- *Base layer: Moisture-wicking clothing worn next to the skin to regulate body temperature and keep hikers dry and comfortable.*
- *Scenic byway: A designated road or highway known for its outstanding natural beauty and recreational opportunities.*
- *Alpine hut: A rustic shelter or lodge located in mountainous regions, offering accommodations and amenities for hikers and climbers.*